# Doing Clinical Healthcare Research

## A Survival Guide

Sarah Winch
Amanda Henderson and
Linda Shields

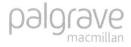

First published 2008 by
PALGRAVE MACMILLAN
Houndmills, Basingstoke, Hampshire RG21 6XS and
175 Fifth Avenue, New York, N.Y. 10010
Companies and representatives throughout the world

PALGRAVE MACMILLAN is the global academic imprint of the Palgrave
Macmillan division of St. Martin's Press, LLC and of Palgrave Macmillan Ltd.
Macmillan® is a registered trademark in the United States, United Kingdom
and other countries. Palgrave is a registered trademark in the European
Union and other countries.

ISBN-13: 978–1–4039–8821–8
ISBN-10: 1–4039–8821–8

This book is printed on paper suitable for recycling and made from fully
managed and sustained forest sources. Logging, pulping and manufacturing
processes are expected to conform to the environmental regulations of the
country of origin.

A catalogue record for this book is available from the British Library.

10   9   8   7   6   5   4   3   2   1
17   16   15   14   13   12   11   10   09   08

Printed and bound in China

W 20.5
A080344

# Contents

**Part three: Collecting data and**
**disseminating findings**

# List of tables and figures

## ▶ Tables

## ▶ Figures

# Acknowledgements

Our work in establishing a research culture in the clinical service sector has shaped the character of this book and we sincerely hope that it meets the needs of clinicians, administrators, post graduate students and beginning researchers.

We would particularly like to acknowledge the support of current and former colleagues in Australia. Executive members of the nursing service at the Princess Alexandra Hospital have been particularly helpful including the former Executive Directors of Nursing, Ms Joy Vickerstaff, Ms Pauline Ross and the current incumbent Ms Veronica Casey.

Mrs Kerri Holzhauser generously provided assistance with two chapters and Mr Brandon Winch has come to our aid with graphic design. Ms Letitia Burridge, *The Journal of Advanced Nursing, The Journal of Clinical Nursing* and *The Queensland Nursing Council* have generously provided material for inclusion in the book.

Ms Catherine James at the Queen Elizabeth II Jubilee Hospital and Professor Debra Creedy at the Faculty of Health, Griffith University, both provided early encouragement to undertake the project. At the University of Queensland, postgraduate students in the School of Social Science helped shaped the flow and content of the ethics chapters and Dr Anne Pisarski from the School of Business provided wisdom on the 'politics' of organizational research.

Our colleagues at The Centaur Memorial Fund for Nurses contributed much enthusiasm and encouragement, particularly Mrs Lyn Chambers, Ms Pixie Annat and Mrs Joy Wilson.

Internationally, we would like to thank the University of Hull, Faculty of Health and Social Care and our publishers Lynda Thompson and Sarah Lodge from Palgrave Macmillan who have provided excellent advice on the organization and production of the book. Many thanks also to Jon Reed previously of Palgrave Macmillan who encouraged the initial concept of rather different style of book on clinical research.

Finally, to our families for their good humour and patience. Not only has this one arrived but we are planning the next!

Sarah Winch, Amanda Henderson and Linda Shields

# About the authors

Dr Sarah Winch, Professor Amanda Henderson and Professor Linda Shields all received their research training in Australia and have collectively been contributing to the clinical research literature for over a decade.

In 2002 Dr Sarah Winch and Professor Amanda Henderson created the Nursing Practice Development Unit at the Princess Alexandra Hospital in Brisbane, Queensland Australia. Mrs Kerri Holzhauser, who has co-authored two chapters, works as a Nurse Researcher in the Emergency Department at the Princess Alexandra Hospital. This hospital was the first to receive 'Magnet' designation in the Southern Hemisphere.

Dr Sarah Winch is Nursing Director, Research, at the Princess Alexandra Hospital and has experience in creating and sustaining research outcomes in busy tertiary environments. Her academic training is in sociology and she holds an adjunct senior lectureship in the School of Social Science at the University of Queensland. In this role she teaches social science students health sociology and research ethics and assists them to access clinical populations. Sarah also has a background in the establishment and management of community and aged care health facilities and is an active researcher in the field of ethics and evidence-based practice.

Dr Amanda Henderson is Nursing Director, Education, at the Princess Alexandra Hospital and holds a Professorial title at Griffith University, Queensland. Her academic training is in science and the sociology of science, with a particular interest in how the context of care shapes what is understood about health. She has been instrumental in the implement-ation of innovative models of clinical learning and education and the development of evidence-based clinical teaching and learning processes. She is presently involved in promoting learning opportunities in clinical practice through the development of communities of engagement with all stakeholders.

Linda Shields is Professor of Nursing and Director of Research in the Faculty of Health and Social Care at the University of Hull in England, and is Honorary Professor in the Department of Paediatrics and Child Health at the University of Queensland, Brisbane, Australia. Linda's research focuses on the care of children and families in health services, health in developing countries and the history of nursing. As Director of Research, she has prepared the faculty for the Research Assessment Exercise, a major part of funding in UK universities. Her research is largely quantitative, and she has an interest in ethics, especially in regard to children. She has a small clinical load in a paediatric post-operative recovery unit, and she teaches both nursing and medical students.

Mrs Kerri Holzhauser is a Nurse Researcher in the Emergency Department for Queensland Health's Southern Area Health Service Emergency Department Clinical Network. Kerri is also an Adjunct Research Fellow with the Research Centre for Clinical Practice Innovation at Griffith University Gold Coast. She is currently undertaking doctoral studies looking at one organization's application process for the Magnet Recognition Program©. She has experience as a principal and associate investigator on a variety of clinical research projects and has developed effective strategies to enable the projects to run smoothly.

# Introduction

Despite the very best intentions of the clinical professions and the growth in the academic sector, research into clinical practice has been slow to develop momentum. Doing clinical research is hard graft and involves drawing together two very different sectors (the practice and academic setting) to provide an outcome that is meaningful for both. Frequently, this has been the task of an individual researcher or a team from one sector with a superficial involvement from the other. This parsimonious approach to clinical research risks producing research findings that have little meaning or value for the clinical sector, or a mass of data that has no ability to describe, explain or predict clinical practice.

This small volume comes from years of experience in initiating, supporting, conducting and completing through to publication stage, research projects in busy health care environments. We have observed the difficulties that researchers from all disciplines, and at all levels of expertise, have faced. Some projects have flourished and some have floundered, wasting resources and the good will of all those involved. Many projects have been completed but never published and those that made it into print were not read or incorporated into practice. This begs a number of questions: (1) Why put yourself through this (either as a researcher or clinical supporter)? (2) Why do some projects succeed and others fail? (3) How do I get academics or clinical administrators on side? (4) As a healthcare administrator, what can I do to make the clinical setting 'research friendly'?

In this book we provide answers to these questions by focussing on how to project manage your research, and if you are a healthcare administrator how to build practice environments that are conducive to research. This is not a research methods text; you won't find any chapters on sampling or statistics! If you do need help in this area, we suggest you find an academic adviser to help you narrow your research question, select the appropriate method and plan how to conduct your research in terms of data collection, analysis and publication. There are already many excellent volumes available that can support you in this area including Parahoo (2006). What has been missing amongst research texts is guidance on how to actually get research happening successfully in busy clinical environments, an outline of the processes needed to operationalize your projects.

If you are an academic, you will learn how to approach healthcare service providers and gain their support. If you are reading this as a senior administrator, you will learn how to create an environment that attracts research and reduces some of the barriers that would-be clinical researchers face. While many healthcare administrators want to establish a research culture, there is not a lot of advice on how to create an environment where research, critical thinking and enquiry can flourish.

## ► How this book can help!

This book has been designed to be informative, easy to use, accessible and above all practical. In Chapter 1 we show how you can gain entry to organizations if you are an outsider; or how to find your way around them if you are an employee. We explain the importance of securing a champion and a sponsor, and selling your research idea. In Chapter 2 we consider the complex area of research ethics and help you systematically identify the ethical aspects of your research. Tips for conducting cross-cultural research both in your own country and abroad are detailed in Chapter 3. In Chapter 4, we show you how to write a master proposal that you can use for a multitude of purposes including ethics and funding applications. Next, in Chapter 5, we show you how to identify, access and recruit your participants. In Chapter 6 we examine how to maximize participation in your study and present tips and tricks for getting clinical staff motivated in your research. Then in Chapter 7 we show you how to collect your data by using a variety of planning and tracking documents. In Chapter 8 we consider the challenges of working data and show you how to organize quantitative and qualitative data. Disseminating findings is the critical final component of doing research. In Chapter 9 we share a variety of tips from how to present at unit meetings to writing press releases and getting published!

Finally in Chapter 10 we provide advice on how to shape your research agenda and manage the risks associated with these activities.

## ► Reference

Parahoo, K. (2006). *Nursing Research: Principles, Process and Issues*. Palgrave Macmillan, Basingstoke, UK.

# Part one
# Preparing your research

# Chapter one

# Overcoming organizational barriers: getting into and around healthcare organizations

*Sarah Winch and Amanda Henderson*

## ► Contents

- ▷ The healthcare organization: maximizing your chances for success
- ▷ Doing due diligence in terms of research
- ▷ Understanding key professional groups and the contribution they can make to your project

Approaching a large healthcare organization as a potential researcher can seem a daunting task. In this chapter we provide guidance on the best ways to proceed and increase your chances for success. We show you how to frame your research in a manner that most healthcare organizations will understand and value. We suggest the range of people who should be involved, and ways to maximize input and commitment from team members. In addition we provide tips on how to deal with the layers of communication involved in getting your project started, and ensuring it proceeds as planned.

Often the best research is an amalgamation of clinical interests, research expertise and passion. Research that is relevant to daily clinical practice will more likely show a return on the investment of time and energy by the health service and therefore be perceived more favourably. It needs to have rigour according to whatever method(s) it uses and has to be sustainable over the length of the project.

Part 1

3

## ▷ The healthcare organization: maximizing your chances for success

In a perceptive insight Manthey (2006) has observed that people working in healthcare organizations are 'FRED'; that is, 'frantically running every day'. We agree! To our knowledge there are no health services that have staff sitting around ready to help stray researchers! Many large hospitals and healthcare services are experiencing staff shortages. There is difficulty in retaining and recruiting staff across all health professional groups. Furthermore, many senior managers change their post every few years. Not surprisingly, the healthcare sector is also subject to ongoing change. In Britain, New Zealand, Canada, United States and Australia restructuring of healthcare services is frequent, changing the way departments operate, reporting lines and services provided (Braithwaite *et al.*, 2005).

The modern healthcare environment is designed to produce high quality health care, quickly and at the lowest cost. Generally healthcare services are run as businesses (whether they are owned by government, charities or private companies). They have business plans and provide services along business lines. Clinical teams are responsible for a particular sector of the business. Senior clinical decisions are made frequently by the medical staff and they often set the research tone and agenda for a clinical unit. They are assisted by business managers who take care of the administrative requirements. Significantly, senior nursing staff control nursing resources and are responsible for the day-to-day smooth functioning of the hospital. Nursing staff provide 24-hour care to the patients and tend to be the eyes and ears of the organization. They can be a very useful source of information on how particular units run and work within a hospital or health service in general. Surrounding these clinical groups are layers of senior managers, business managers, quality and audit staff, and ancillary workers.

It is into this environment that the healthcare researcher has to pitch their research idea and capture the imagination of those who are going to support the research through its many stages to completion. Our role is to show you how to move through these stages within what may be an unsympathetic healthcare environment and share tips and tricks that will help you succeed.

Knowing the type of environment that you are going to approach will help you pitch your research project in the best possible manner. If you already work within the organization then you will have some inside knowledge on whom to contact in the organization and the type of service provision the hospital is known for and wishes to promote. If you are coming from outside, you will need to obtain this information so that you can be sure that you are approaching the organization that potentially will have the most interest in your research.

While the health service environment is busy and frequently stretched to the limit, most organizations are striving to do the very best for their patients. Many administrators are impressed by the idea of excellence and the creation of knowledge that can really make a difference for patients. In the United States those hospitals that promote nursing research and education through the Magnet Services Recognition Program are able to recruit and retain their nursing staff and reduce patient mortality (Aiken *et al.* 2001). In our experience many, if not all, hospitals are generally happy to support research endeavours, as long as it suits their core business direction and needs. What they are often not sure about is what is involved and how they can give the best support.

Let us look at two scenarios. The first is a nurse academic (Dr Jane) who is keen to start her research programme following graduation from her Doctor of Philosophy. Jane is looking to build up her 'track record'. A track record refers to the amount of research grant money that an individual or team has won in a competitive environment (the inputs for research), and the amount of publications that the individual or team have following the completion of the research (the outputs that show they have completed the work to a high standard). For academics of all disciplines and clinical researchers, building their track record is critical to their success. To achieve this, clinical researchers need to access clinical populations. Jane has moved to the university to take up her post and she knows no one at the local hospital, a busy 700-bed medical and surgical service provider that is also a major trauma centre. We shall call this facility the City Metropolitan Hospital.

The second example involves a senior clinical nurse (James) working at the oncology unit at the City Metropolitan Hospital. James has just completed his masters degree and has been given the research portfolio for the ward. Both of these individuals, one from inside the organization, and one from outside, have to try and progress their research interests and endeavours in a way that is going to be sustainable and useful for the organization. Both of these researchers need to find common ground that is going to have traction with the organization, be that at a broad strategic level or within a clinical unit. They need to find out what type of research the organization wants to support. The following checklist provides a starting point for discovering information about your target organization, be that as an employee or a visiting researcher.

---

### Check List: Finding out about organizations from the outside

**Doing due diligence in terms of research planning**

The following information should be readily available from the health service website or the facility Annual Report:

- ☑ Size and type of organization (tax payer funded or private)
- ☑ Name of Chief Executive Officer (your first point of contact)
- ☑ Name of Director of Nursing
- ☑ Name of Chief Medical Officer or the Medical Superintendent
- ☑ Name of Chief Allied Health Officer
- ☑ Service profile or case mix
- ☑ Patient profile (gender, age and catchment areas)
- ☑ Organizational Chart (will show the structure of the organization, senior officer responsibilities and portfolios, and reporting relationships)
- ☑ Strategic Directions Statement (will tell you where the organization is planning to be)

---

In addition, the following documents are useful because they give you an idea of what research is already being conducted in an organization. Not all facilities publish such reports and they are not always available to people who work outside of the organization. However, it is worth trying to request them, perhaps at your first meeting with a senior administrator. Jane and James now have some broad information that is going to help

---

### Check List: Useful internal documents that help you frame your research

- ☑ Research Plan (whole of Organization)
- ☑ Annual Research Reports
- ☑ Nursing Plan
- ☑ Nursing Research Plan
- ☑ Senior Nursing Administrators, their roles and responsibilities
- ☑ The organizational research register
- ☑ Ethics Committee Annual Reports

---

them frame their research in a language and context that is meaningful for the organization. For example, the research report will show the research directions of the organization and the type and intensity of the research that is already happening. This will give you an indication of how much capacity the facility has for supporting your research.

As an employee of the organization, James will certainly be able to access the following documents.

> ### Check List: Finding out about organizations from the inside (at the unit level)
>
> ☑ Current Business Plan
> ☑ Case mix
> ☑ Staffing ratios
> ☑ Multi-disciplinary interests
> ☑ Existing Research programs and projects

## ! Hot Tip: Creating a research or practice development plan

Increasingly, many organizations are developing research or practise development plans. These can be multidisciplinary or focused on one aspect of a whole organization such as the nursing service. If you work in a health service that does not have one – how about suggesting that one is created? The plan needs to be flexible enough to respond to opportunities but direct enough to shape the research direction of the facility. In Chapter 10 we show you how to successfully meld health services needs with opportunities.

## ▶ Getting 'legs' for your research idea: the hook and the heart

It is important from the outset to prepare your approach to the healthcare facility by clarifying your research question and framing it in a language and form that healthcare organizations can understand. It is helpful to demonstrate clearly the return on the investment (time, energy or money) that the health service is going to provide.

**Part 1**

Undertaking and supporting research involves a substantial commitment from all stakeholders, particularly if the results are to be meaningful and inform policy and practice. For your project to be successful it needs to be consistent with the interest and direction of how the health facility delivers their service; it needs to get 'legs' of its own that will carry it through the organization when you are not there to talk it up!

In our experience you need to create two aspects to your research, a hook, a particular issue of significance, that will attract the management support that you need and a heart, that is, the meaning or value embedded in what you are trying to achieve, that will attract the clinicians! The degree of significance of the question to the management team or the local clinical staff will form the hook for their support.

Invariably health facilities will invest time, effort, energy and commitment if they are of the impression that the research will inform or facilitate their core business and if the findings will be useful in making informed changes to the health service. They need to see a return for their investment that will make their support worthwhile. Think about your project – what is it going to deliver for the organization? These deliverables may be broad such as increased staff satisfaction or narrow such as direct cost savings.

A direct appeal to patient care issues or staff development will form the heart of the project that will attract and sustain the interest of the clinicians and hopefully the participants in the research. While many patients are altruistic and like to participate for the greater good of science and knowledge development in general, also identifying a potential direct benefit is always useful. This process is used to enrol patients in clinical trials where they have a chance to receive an experimental drug that may improve their condition. In a recent study conducted by Pisarski *et al.* (2006), staff were motivated to participate because the intervention component of the project had the potential to assist them to improve their management skills. They were keen to become better managers and this study appealed to them because of the direct benefit that they could experience.

### ▶ Tips for developing useful research questions

While an organization may have strategic goals for developing research, there is often a limited body of practice knowledge that can assist the facility in reaching these goals. It is important to approach an organization (either externally or internally) with a research proposal that is direct enough to demonstrate what the topic is and what the outcomes will be but with enough flexibility to incorporate further refinement by senior management and clinical staff.

We said at the start of this chapter that the best research is a blend of passion, expertise and organizational interest. The passion that the researcher has for their topic drives them to overcome barriers and succeed. Postgraduate research training provides the expertise that the researcher needs. The trick now is to blend the researcher's passion for their topic with the healthcare facilities' direction.

Thus, researchers internal and external to the organization need to meld their research expertise with the direction of the facility. This can be in terms of method or subject area. For example, Jane, our new academic, has expertise in discharge planning for gynaecology patients. The City Metropolitan Hospital does not have a gynaecology unit but is concerned with the discharge and readmission of patients in its orthopaedic unit. Jane decides to broaden her focus and offers to repeat her research and test her discharge planning tool with a new patient population. Meanwhile James, as an employee of the organization, has access to the incident and error data that is happening on his unit. This is a useful source to inform research questions. It has immediate appeal to supervisors and colleagues as it addresses issues related to patient safety.

## Check List: Framing your project to get traction: the hook and the heart

- ☑ Consistent with core business
- ☑ Recruitment and retention: across the spectrum of the workforce
- ☑ Patient flow
- ☑ Patient safety
- ☑ Complex clinical topics – facilitating dialogue across multidisciplinary approach
- ☑ Saving money – economic evaluations very useful

▶ **Understanding key professional groups and the contribution they can make to your project**

Medical research is the most common type of research undertaken in large clinical facilities. This type of research tends to have a very narrow clinical

Part 1

focus as befits the discipline of medicine itself. Medical officers (residents, registrars or consultants) are significant gatekeepers to patients and are important stakeholders to get on side in any research project or planned research programme. One of the common difficulties that we have experienced is that many medical officers, particularly those in Australia, have had limited exposure to research traditions and methods other than the 'Randomised Control Trial'. In addition, they are absolutely time poor. If you are using a social science–derived research methodology, you will need to convince them that the method is sound. This can be achieved by demonstrating the value to them in terms of patient care, or staff satisfaction. Keeping team members happy is in the interest of most senior clinical staff!

Understanding nursing takes a different set of skills. This is very much a relationship-based, patient-focused, oral culture (Horder 2004). This is a group that may take some time to respond to emails! It is also a very hierarchical profession which means multiple meetings and 'sign offs'. Like medical staff, nurses are busy, so you need a strong hook to get their attention. In our experience, we have found nurses educated through the tertiary system to a baccalaureate standard (as most are in Australia) have a broader understanding of research informed by social science traditions.

### ▶ Champions and sponsors

Researchers working within and those working outside the organization need a champion and a sponsor. Champions are people who are often senior in the organization who are going to speak up for your project. In large organizations, decisions about research may be made by committees or at unit meetings where the researcher is not present, with the decision-makers referring to a short appraise of your topic. A champion is someone who shares the passion for your topic and is prepared to speak up it in the face of criticism or even smooth your path across some of the barriers you may face.

You also need to find a sponsor. A sponsor is the person who is going to steer you through the organizational processes to ensure that your project succeeds. They will actually do some of the work for you by getting in contact with people inside the organization, obtaining forms, finding out when various groups of people pertinent to the success of your research meet or the times that the ethics committee meets.

The challenge for researchers within the organization is gathering momentum and enthusiasm for the research topic within the clinical field in unison with sufficient academic guidance and monetary support. Below

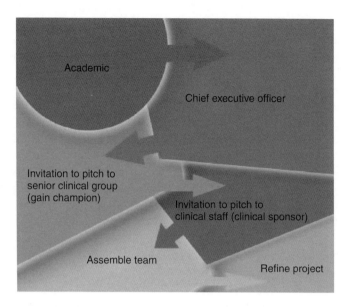

Academic

Chief executive officer

Invitation to pitch to
senior clinical group
(gain champion)

Invitation to pitch to
clinical staff (clinical sponsor)

Assemble team

Refine project

**Figure 1.1**   *Flow chart for approaching organizations from the outside*

is a flow chart to help guide you through process of getting support for
your project from healthcare facilities.

### Reference/steering groups

Some projects may benefit from a reference or steering group. These
are particularly useful for large projects that involve a number of clinical
areas or disciplines. This group should consist of expert professionals and
stakeholders who provide direct oversight of the research from the organizational perspective. They are not part of the research team as such but
often have a vested interest in knowing the findings, as usually this will
have a major influence on how they pursue their business. The steering
group 'ensures the research is on track' in terms of progress within the
organization and meeting organizational goals.

### Linking clinicians and academics

While clinicians may have an interest, beginning knowledge and access
to internal data to progress clinically relevant research, that can generate useful findings for clinical practice, their projects can generally be
improved when they link with research-trained academics. Not all academics conduct research, a few have focussed their career on teaching,
curriculum development and university administration. It is important to

Part 1

link with an academic who is prepared at a doctoral level (i.e. an academic who holds the qualification of Doctor of Philosophy) and is research active. This will ensure that the academic is trained in research methods and processes, publication of findings and applying for research funds.

The engagement between the academic and their institution, and health-care worker and their facility can be fraught with issues that can trap the unsuspecting clinician (or academic). The ideal is a close relationship between the clinicians and the academics at many levels. The challenge is to create a situation that ensures that all partner's goals have been reached. Many senior administrators have established links with local nursing academe. If you are a clinician who is hoping to progress a research project, you need to find out where these links are and who is the link person within your organization. If you are a senior nurse administrator looking at fostering a research culture in your organization then you need to establish these links, perhaps through a 'Visiting Scholar' programme (more on this in Chapter 10).

### Developing research projects that suit clinicians and academics

While the achievements of the research can be synonymous and beneficial to both organizations, the needs of both are rarely the same. This issue needs to be raised and clarified, and a commitment can be made to address the needs of both the clinician and the researcher. For this reason, it is not unusual for the proposed research project to develop over many meetings through a number of months. The initial discussions between parties may be slow as both parties require an understanding of each other's needs, their reasons for becoming involved and what each party hopes to achieve. It is important in these early stages that the process remains fluid. This fluidity will assist in ensuring the expression of many ideas and issues. It also facilitates the appropriate membership of the team when the research 'starts to develop legs' because members who are disinterested in the process and/or the area of study will drop out.

### ▶ The team: identifying and accessing relevant players

Research is a lengthy process and enthusiasm for your project can some-times falter (and that is just from your perspective let alone the wider group who are going to support and enable your research). Whether you are an individual or part of a team it is important that there is a mechanism that assists in your continued application to the project. Keeping things 'rolling along' is paramount. Despite this it is common to witness individuals and teams flagging when they are halfway through the project because issues relating to clarification of the research question, or insufficient exploration of the research area in general prior to commencement, result in changes during data collection. While minor 'hiccups' are congruent with research in the 'real world', careful planning of the question (in line with organizational needs or interests), involvement and regular communication with all the players can ideally limit major 'mid-stream' changes that can curtail the impact and rigour of the findings.

When constructing a team, it is beneficial to identify 'experts' who are familiar with your area of research. Discussing your research with these experts can give you important feedback. Such players can advise and avert possible 'dead ends' when you embark on the research process. It is worthwhile to access expertise in a number of different areas, including the content, practice area and also the research method. Seeking out assistance can be through local knowledge of interested people or through identifying an expert who has a known track record (identifiable through the published literature). For individual researchers, these experts can become informal assistants to your project (however, it is important that they are acknowledged or, depending on their contribution, even become an author of the final work). Potential team members will join depending on how relevant the project is to their capabilities, research directions or the opportunity to develop new skills. Factors such as time and other commitments will also determine their ability to participate in the research.

### Specific considerations for teams

It pays to make sure that you have the right team for your project from the start. This can help you avoid some of the more common pitfalls later on in the project. Team members need to have a blend of clinical and research experience. Of paramount importance is that the chief or principal investigator(s) need to have significant research experience expertise; that is, experience in planning, conducting and completing research within a healthcare facility.

Who to include in the rest of the team is rarely clear-cut but will relate to the study being undertaken. There is a reasonable published literature on teams that specify which personality types should be included in the team to get the best outcome. If you have the luxury of doing this then by all means do so. For the purposes of operationalizing your research project, that is actually getting the project going you need to include a blend of academics and clinicians who will facilitate the processes and

Part 1

conduct of the research. While a number of 'innovator' and 'creator' type personalities are essential through the initial development and conceptualization of the project, too many of these individuals towards the latter stages of the research can steer the whole project off the rails! Getting the best team means getting a mixture of individuals who have a good complement of skills.

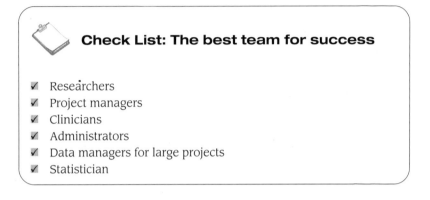

**Check List: The best team for success**

☑ Researchers
☑ Project managers
☑ Clinicians
☑ Administrators
☑ Data managers for large projects
☑ Statistician

The leader of the team (the Principal or Chief Investigator) should specify roles for each team member; for example: Who will draft the initial proposal? Who will review it? And, by what date or time? When the project outline is written, specify who will recruit subjects, collect and input the data, analyse and write the first draft of the report. In intervention studies clarification is needed about who is going to conduct the intervention and who will organize the research subjects to take part.

The Chief Investigator also needs to communicate with the facility administrators to ensure that everyone is happy with the direction that the project is taking. If you have convened a steering group, make sure this meets regularly. Once everyone has agreed on the direction of the research and on the resources and processes required (be those financial, in kind, or disruption to the clinical area), then the Chief Investigator secures support in writing. These approval letters are needed for future grants and ethics applications. They are also useful when senior administrators change (and they do quite frequently) as a record of what has been agreed to.

## ! Hot Tip: Effective team work

Effective teams explain and delegate the contributions of all members.

## Check List: Academic and clinician capabilities

| Academic(s) | Clinician and clinical administrator |
|---|---|
| ☑ Expert knowledge in research methods and design | ☑ Expert clinical knowledge of the patient population |
| ☑ Knowledge of the literature or ability to rapidly acquire that knowledge | ☑ Expert knowledge of the organization or the ability to rapidly acquire that knowledge |
| ☑ Knowledge of how the literature can influence the research question | ☑ Expert knowledge on staffing and staffing patterns |
| ☑ Ability to derive a research question from a clinical problem area | ☑ Ability to gain medical support |
| ☑ Experience in data collection and storage | ☑ Ability to identify and recruit appropriate participants into studies |
| ☑ Experience in ethics applications | ☑ Knowledge of the organizations policies on ethics applications (cut-off dates for submission, resource approvals) |
| ☑ Experience in data analysis and drawing conclusions and findings from data | ☑ Ability to provide some type of support in kind for the academic such as use of a telephone, filing cabinet or desk |
| ☑ Ability to publish findings in the relevant journals | ☑ Ability to put the findings into practice within the organization |

## Critical capabilities for successful research teams: academics and clinicians

Academics and clinicians provide different but complementary strengths and areas of expertise to the team. Nurses have a well-deserved, excellent reputation as research participant recruiters, data collectors and data managers, particularly in medical research. This is because of their excellent patient skills, understanding of the ward environment and ability to follow through. For a true partnership, the nurse can bring these skills to the team and most significantly contribute to the actual research question and develop a body of knowledge that will inform nursing practice.

While the clinician is invaluable, they probably have the least reason to be interested – as this work is not something that they generally aspire to (if they did, they would not be clinicians!). For this reason, the academic may need to keep clinicians motivated throughout the duration of the research. The following checklist outlines the strengths that are generally associated with academics and clinicians, and how these skills can contribute to the overall success of the project. This division is not always clear-cut as some experienced clinical researchers working within hospitals can provide both the skills of the academic and the clinician.

## ▶ 'Getting started' making contact and keeping people on-side

### Starting the research

It is a good idea to start your discussions around a broad research question or area that allows everyone to have some input, according to the interests of each member. You need to get agreement from your team to develop a research proposal that everyone agrees is worthwhile to progress. However, care needs to be taken that the project does not become unwieldy or unachievable because everyone wants to have their say in the research!

The next step in the process is to review the proposal to identify those people this work may affect. This may include specific groups of staff that may potentially be threatened by the research. For example, the implications from the research may significantly affect the jurisdiction of a group. Consider carefully the potential impact of the research on patients, staff and the facility in general. Ideally, people representing these interests have been included in your discussions or on your team from the beginning;

however, research can metamorphose and take a different look to what was initially proposed. If you have convened a stakeholder group or reference group, they will assist here and be able to give advice on how to lessen any potential adverse outcomes. In a recent example we were aware of a group of nurse unit managers who felt uncomfortable about a project exploring particular information needs of staff. Their discomfort was based on the assumption that they must be inadequate if staff reported not having sufficient preparation and knowledge to undertake a particular activity within their unit. Such research has the potential to be confronting because it has the capacity (although not necessarily the intention) to measure the behaviour of others in a negative way. In this case it was important to involve the nurse unit managers in the research to allow them to make a contribution. Following their input, another arm that identifies barriers to communication for nurse unit managers was added to the study.

Now you are ready to use the Master proposal format discussed in Chapter 4. By addressing the criteria in this template, you will have all the requirements necessary to obtain ethics approval and complete funding applications. In addition, summary versions of the plan make great communication tools when trying to build your team and communicate with staff.

---

### ! Hot tip: Maintaining momentum during the ethics process

Take care not to lose momentum during ethics approval. This can be a slow process so maintain the communication channels. While the research itself cannot commence without ethics approval, use this time to establish the systems and processes that need to be in place during the project.

---

### Keeping people informed

Once you have ethical approval, the data collection can commence. While healthcare facilities vary in size, complexity and routines, they are all invariably busy. This has clear implications for researchers who need to have a communication strategy in mind from the start of the project. A first step is to be clear about what is required from the clinical setting. If you are wise, you will have a clinician or administrator on your team who is able to communicate with the targeted clinical area. Nevertheless, whether the project investigates staff, patients or carers, the team needs to be clear about what will be happening and what is involved. For example, when, how and who from your team will be collecting data. It is important that everybody is comfortable with the additional activity that results from the research. Staff in healthcare facilities are used to a range of different people entering and leaving the environment without always knowing the purpose of the visitors to the area. This is particularly the case if a person has a uniform and carrying a folder or official looking material. The members of the team should always ask permission to enter the area and link with the person-in-charge and also inform the present team leader and relevant others about what is happening.

This needs to happen every time the team enters the facility. This is not because the efforts of the team or management have been poor, but rather in the dynamic complex environments staff readily sort out the 'need to know' from the 'nice to know'. Some staff have no interest in research and consequently do not recall ever being advised about it. Others will comment that they 'heard something'! They will rarely be proactive in the dissemination of the information – rather they choose to act when 'the time comes'. That time is when the researcher makes contact with the person-in-charge and ideally they arrange a meeting to manage the logistics. This meeting is very important to establish a positive 'tone' so that the research can proceed as smoothly as possible.

**Following organizational protocols**
Each healthcare facility has a suite of protocols that all staff and official visitors (such as external researchers) have to follow. This ranges from where to park, use of telephones, to basic security measures such as identification badges and assembly points in case of a fire. In any clinical setting it is essential that research staff wear an identification badge. When entering the area, the researcher(s) should introduce themselves to who is in charge in the immediate area and encourage the person-in-charge to introduce them to other staff. A brief but comprehensive plain language explanation should be given so that staff on the clinical unit understand what is going to occur.

Ideally, all the staff should already be familiar with the project. However repeatedly, we find that no matter how prolific communication has been, there are always staff members who have not heard about the project. Or, they have 'sort of' heard about it but didn't really understand what it meant in terms of their day-to-day work schedule. From our experience entering the clinical area needs to be well planned and certainly not undertaken in a hurry. ALWAYS leave plenty of time! Other priorities may overtake your appointment with the person-in-charge who still has to respond to clinical needs. Don't be discouraged if you have a few false starts as investing this time at the beginning is worthwhile because on each subsequent visit you can pick up threads from this first visit (as someone will usually remember something)! All of this contact can significantly contribute to the positive feelings and attitudes that clinical staff develop towards your project.

## ! Hot Tip: Dealing with preconceived notions/ assumptions and negative views about research

Unfortunately, there may be staff that hold negative views about research being conducted in their area. For many staff their experience of research has not been positive but rather of the 'grab and run' variety. That is, the researchers came in, collected the data and took it away to be analysed with no feedback or involvement with the clinical area. Thankfully, this is not common now but there can still be prejudices in the clinical area because of this former practice.

There is a greater attraction for clinicians to participate in or support research if the researcher is able to provide something for them, for example, an intervention focused around teaching sessions for the staff or feedback in the form of statistics about changes to a practice. In our experience interventions focused on teaching conflict management or providing clinical supervision for staff are positively received. These are viewed as tangible benefits that encourage involvement.

### Starting the communication process

Of key importance in any large, complex organization is the way that you are going to communicate what you are doing and keep everyone up to date about your project and more importantly onside.

You need to develop a plan that addresses the information needs of all the members of the research team so that they are clear about their responsibilities and clinical staff in the areas where the research is being undertaken to ensure their continued support. The plan should also address how you are going to facilitate timely progress reports to ethics committees and funding bodies.

The communication plan needs to be agreed to by all the members of the research team. Once this agreement has been reached, then all

Part 1

relevant personnel associated with the project are clearly informed prior to the beginning and subsequently as the project progresses. Accordingly, staff have time to plan for the periods when they may have considerable involvement in the project. This potentially enhances support by the team members and clarifies ambiguities around the research. It is not unusual to hear staff members and/or participants commenting that 'they heard something about some research'; however, nothing has been forthcoming, indicating that it has either stalled or possibly even finished without staff being informed.

The following template developed by Mrs Kerri Holzhauser can be used to plan your communication efforts in a systematic manner.

Communication that is timely and regular needs to occur to all members of the research team so that they are clear about their contribution to the research. At each stage of the research project (as detailed in the planning phase) emails should be sent to all staff providing an update on activities.

**Table 1.1**   *Planning a Communication strategy*

| Communication strategy | | | |
|---|---|---|---|
| Goal: Gain clinical support for the research project and maximize participation for successful completion of project | | | |
| *Target groups* | *Marketing tools available* | *Key issues* | *Evaluation* |
| • Executive management<br>• Divisional directors<br>• Clinical managers<br>• Clinical staff | • Official memos both snail mail and email<br>• Flyers<br>• Newsletter<br>• Consolidated circular<br>• PowerPoint presentation<br>• Direct communication<br>• Forums (internal) | • Clarify the project<br>• Early identification of problems/issues of project to ensure appropriate solutions created<br>• Time required for participation within project will require executive support<br>• Disseminate the involvement required during project | • Tracking knowledge of project within the facility<br>• Monitor feedback at various stages of the project |

## ▶ Summary

In this chapter we have considered how to frame your question so that there is a hook and a heart that grabs the attention of clinical or academic partners. We have reviewed a number of factors that will be critical to the success of your project including the use of a detailed communication plan. We have summarized these key points in the following check list.

---

### Check List: Summary for project preparation success

☑ Champion found amongst senior staff
☑ Sponsor available
☑ Research topics address organizational needs or research priorities (hook)
☑ Funding or resources are available or will be applied for
☑ Academic partner(s) have necessary research experience
☑ Clinical staff have a broad understanding and developed a commitment to the research topic and therefore likely to co-operate in data collection
☑ Clinical staff (medical and nursing are committed to the project)
☑ Communication plan developed

---

You are now ready to consider the ethical and cultural implications of your research (Chapters 2 and 3) and how to construct a master research plan (Chapter 4).

## ▶ References

Aiken, L.H., Clarke, S.P., Sloane, D., Sochalski, J.A., Busse, R., Clarke, H., Giovannetti, P., Hunt, J., Rafferty, A.M. and Shamian, J. (2001). Nurses' reports on hospital care in five countries. *Health Affairs*, 20: 43–51.
Braithwaite, J., Westbrook, J.I. and Iedema, R. (2005). Restructuring as gratification. *Journal of the Royal Society of Medicine*, 98(12): 542–4.
Horder, W. (2004). Reading and not reading in professional practice. *Qualitative Social Work*, 3(3): 297–311.

Part 1

Manthey, M. (2006). Relationship-based care: customized primary nursing . . . *Creative Nursing: A Journal of Values, Issues, Experience and Collaboration*, 12(1): 4–9.

Pisarski, A., Brook, C., Bohle, P., Gallois, C., Watson, B. and Winch, S. (2006). Extending a model of shiftwork tolerance. *Chronobiology*, 23(6): 1363–1377.

# Chapter two

# Ethical considerations: informed consent and protecting vulnerable populations

*Linda Shields and Sarah Winch*

## ▶ Contents

▷ The history and role of ethics committees
▷ An overview of ethical principles as they relate to research
▷ The nature of 'informed consent'
▷ Ethical issues for different groups
▷ Dealing with unethical behaviour
▷ The difference between privacy, confidentiality and anonymity
▷ Protecting research subjects

Previously, as a researcher you will have been concerned with refining your research question and finding the correct method to provide answers to your problem. Now you will need to consider the ethical implications of your project. How will you maintain the dignity of your research subjects? Are there any cultural beliefs or customs you need to respect? Does your research involve people with impaired capacity such as people with an illness that causes cognitive impairment or very young children? If so, how will you as a researcher address these issues to the satisfaction of all parties concerned? Nearly all research that is conducted will require formal approval from a research ethics committee. This provides a form of protection for you as a researcher, the organization where the research is to be conducted and most importantly, your research subjects. In this chapter we explain why this is necessary and in the next chapter we tell you how to go about it!

## ▶ The role of ethics committees

In many countries, for example, the Nordic countries, Australia and the United Kingdom, there is a long tradition of Human Research Ethics Committees based in healthcare institutions and universities. In health services, two types of ethics committees exist. The first examines ethical dilemmas which arise in practice, and their deliberations and conclusions are used to guide decision-making when an ethical dilemma arises. These are clinical ethics committees and deal with matters quite separate to research ethics committees. The second type of ethics committee is the Human Research Ethics Committee (HREC), the 'watch dog' for the ethical conduct of research. Research ethics committees are constituted according to certain rules and principles based on the Helsinki Declaration. In Australia, the United Kingdom, the United States, New Zealand, Canada and many other developed countries, as well as many developing countries for example Indonesia and Thailand, most hospital and health services will have access to a research ethics committee. In addition all universities have research ethics committees. In some cases where the researcher is an employee of the university or a student, ethics approval will be needed from both committees.

A research ethics committee comprises generally a lay man and woman, a minister of religion, a lawyer and several experienced medical researchers from a variety of backgrounds. Many also include a pharmacology expert as a great deal of the work of research ethics committees is related to approving drug trials by pharmaceutical companies.

## ▶ The history of ethical approval for research

Ironically, Germany was probably the first country to have a code of ethics for research experiments in the early 20th century (Sauerteig 2000), but the notion of ethical review of research by a committee arose from the atrocities that took place during the Second World War. In 1945, at the end of the Second World War, the liberating forces were shocked to find that prisoners in some of the concentration camps had been used as guinea pigs in a wide range of medical experiments. Many were fruitless, gratuitous experiments with no real purpose; others had a purpose, for example, to see how extreme cold affects the human body. In all cases, the people on whom the experiments were carried out were forced to participate against their will, under egregious conditions and were killed once the experiments were completed (Shields and Twycross 2003). At the Nuremberg Trials some of the perpetrators were called to account (some escaped before the trials began) but the result of the medical trials was a code for the ethical conduct of research, the 'Nuremberg Code' (Annas and Grodin 1992).

The tenets of the Nuremberg Code were strengthened by the World Medical Association's Helsinki Code in 1964, a statement of ethical principles developed by the World Medical Association to 'provide guidance to physicians and other participants in medical research involving human subjects' (Para 1, Declaration of Helsinki). This includes research on people, identifiable human material or identifiable data. The Declaration includes principles on safeguarding research subjects, informed consent, minimizing risk and adhering to an approved research plan/protocol. We will consider the practical implications of each of these later in the chapter.

These documents have become the cornerstone of ethical conduct in health and social research where humans are involved as subjects. Later work by governments and lobby groups has seen the development of codes of ethical conduct of research on animals, and most institutions where research using animals occurs usually have a separate animal ethics committee.

## ▶ Adhering to ethical standards

When designing and planning your research project, it is imperative that you maintain ethical standards. Researcher(s) need to demonstrate justice and respect to participants, and describe how they will provide informed consent, and how vulnerable groups will be managed.

### Demonstrating justice and respect

Participation as a research subject should be just; that is, the burdens and benefits of the research should be shared across a number of populations. 'Captive' audiences either literally or figuratively including prisoners, university students and health service employees such as nurses can be subject to over-researching as they are relatively easy to access. If you do want to survey an over researched population then you need to justify how your study is going to add substantially to the body of knowledge. Your research design needs to demonstrate that the selection, recruitment, exclusion and inclusion criteria are fair. The following checklist will help you ensure that you are treating your participants respectfully.

**Part 1**

---

> ### Check List: Demonstrating respect for the wellbeing of all participants
>
> ☑ Describe how you will minimize harm and discomfort (including psychological harm).
> ☑ What are the risks to participants? Is there a possibility they will become upset by telling you their experiences? If so, how will you deal with this?
> ☑ What is the size of these risks?
> ☑ How likely are these risks?

---

**First 'do no harm'!**

One of the most important principles of any healthcare research is non-maleficence, that is, do no harm. A prominent feature of the dreadful experiments in the Nazi concentration camps was the direct harm done to the subjects by the experiments; in other words, they were designed to cause pain. Other experiments have inadvertently resulted in harm to the subjects, for example, the Milgram experiments in 1961–1962 where subjects were instructed to give electric shocks to others as a way of measuring how much obedience to someone in authority influenced how people behaved (in reality, those receiving the shocks were actors who acted in pain when a pretend shock was given to them, but the subjects under examination did not know that). The subjects in these experiments were psychologically traumatized for years afterwards, though the designers of the experiments did not foresee such an effect (Cave and Holm 2003). When the researchers realized that harm was being done to their subjects, they stopped the experiment, but this did not happen until significant harm had been done. Such experiments are, of course, unethical and, obviously, are even more unethical if they are continued after harmful effects are detected.

Drug trials are a common situation where research is stopped if harmful effects are found. However, there are exceptions; for example, in cancer treatment research, chemotherapy can have severe side effects and cause harm to the subjects. However, the trials are continued as the new drug may be the only possible hope of extending the life of the subject; in other words, the person will definitely die without the drugs but has a chance of living if the experimental drug works. So a decision has to be made based on the balance of assessments of benefit, that is, the possibility of a longer life, against the harm of the side effects. However, the converse can occur.

In some cases, drug trials are stopped before the trial is complete because it becomes apparent before the end of the trial that the drug is effective and will benefit people. In these cases, it would be unethical to deprive patients, who are potential recipients, the drug until the trial is complete.

Perhaps the most useful way of describing when to stop a research project is to say that if any undue or unforeseen event or emotion occurs, is prolonged and looks likely to cause a deal of distress and/or harm, then the project should be put on hold. If you as a researcher or an administrator have any concerns regarding the harmful aspects of the research then you seek advice from a research ethics committee member or a senior colleague.

## ▶ Informed consent

One of the central issues of the Nuremberg and subsequent codes is informed consent; in other words, making sure that your subjects, or their advocates, for example parents, care givers or those who hold legal responsibility for the subjects, are happy to participate based on being fully informed of the consequences, risks and benefits.

### Check List: Gaining informed consent

☑  The participant must not be coerced (by withholding treatment or by influencing employment).
☑  The participant must not be induced by monetary payments (although compensation for expenses is acceptable).
☑  Participants must know what is going to happen to them by acting as research subjects; for example: What procedures or tests are involved? How long the survey instrument will take to fill out? And, what will the researcher ask?
☑  The risks of the research should be clearly identified.
☑  The benefits must also be identified; for example: What they will gain – be it payment for the service, compensation for costs incurred, a gift, or satisfaction from acting out of altruism? They also need to know how the project will benefit other people, or the world at large.

### Ethical ways of obtaining informed consent

There are various ways of obtaining informed consent, depending on the project, the subjects and the environment in which the study is taking place. A trial of a new cancer drug for adults will require the consent of the person, while a study of anything to do with infants requires parental consent. However, if a child is old enough to understand what the study is all about, and the benefits and risks – that is, is 'Gillick competent' (explained later in this chapter) – then the child can legally consent for himself/herself. Some ethics committees, though, will still require the parent to consent as well as the child.

A contentious issue for both applicants and those who sit on HRECs relates to how subjects are invited to participate in the study, or how they are recruited. Imagine a nurse is conducting a study about a new wound care treatment, and asks clients at a leg ulcer clinic to agree to be subjects. The clients might think that if they do not take part, the nurse may be upset and give them inferior treatment. They may have a really good relationship with the nurse and agree to participate even though they do not really want to. Conversely, if they do not like the nurse, they may refuse to participate even though they could see benefits for themselves and others from the research.

Ethics committees often demand a process around potential problems of perceived coercion. They talk about 'power gradients' (and this is discussed at length in the ethics literature [Garrard and Dawson 2005]). If the research is to adhere to ethical standards, the researcher(s) need to demonstrate that a process is in place to protect against the subjects' feeling that they must participate. There are a couple of safe and (relatively) easy ways around this. The first is to have someone who is unknown to the potential participants to invite them to take part in the project. A research assistant on the project, a person who does voluntary work in the health facility, or a colleague could be the one who approaches the potential participants, discusses the project with them, gives them the information sheet, asks them to think about whether or not they would like to be involved, and tells them that the 'inviter' will return after a period of time to receive their answer. This can be done by the principal investigator if he/she is unknown to the potential participants. An alternative is an information sheet about the project, with an invitation to participate, given to the potential participants with their admission documentation, or posted to them independently or, perhaps, sent by email.

Another issue in relation to coercion is the timing of recruitment. HRECs will not approve a project that would, for example, recruit subjects who are on their way into the operating theatre and have been given a pre-medication. Recruitment must be done in a place and time that is the least coercive possible.

---

### Check List: Situations when subjects must *not* be recruited

☑ When subjects feel they have no option but to agree
☑ When subjects are too ill or frightened to be able to think through what participation might mean for them
☑ When subjects are harried or hassled into a decision
☑ When subjects think they or their families will be disadvantaged if they do not take part
☑ When subjects are under the influence of medication which would make decision-making difficult, for example, pre-operative medication

---

### Information sheets and consent forms

Information sheets advise potential participants about the research. Consideration needs to be given to when these are given out and the subsequent consent obtained. It is best practice to give potential subjects plenty of time to read and discuss the information sheet. In addition, make sure that the subjects' family are involved in the discussion and decision process. The HREC application will ask you to explain how these procedures are to be handled.

In your research ethics proposal you will need to include a copy of both the information sheet and the consent form. Some HRECs, especially those in health facilities, may want you to provide an information sheet to all staff who come in contact with the research. For example, if your research is in a hospital ward, you will have to provide written information explaining to the staff of the ward what the research is about and which patients are subjects. A copy will be placed in the chart of each subject. Occasionally, you may not want staff to know that you are asking such things. If you have a good reason for excluding staff, explain this in your ethics application, and state that you want to protect your subjects' confidentiality.

A sample information sheet is included in Figure 2.1. It includes all of the items in the following checklist.

Part 1

**WUTHERING HEIGHTS HOSPITAL
DINGO STREET, LONDON**

Information Sheet

Dear Patient,

I am conducting research at the Wuthering Heights Hospital. I am studying wound care, to see how having a wound can affect your life. In this way, the care of patients in hospitals can possibly be improved.

I am asking patients in this hospital if they would consider helping with the study. If you agree, it will mean we will have a discussion about some aspects of wound care, which will take about half-an-hour, and this will be audio-taped.

All information is strictly confidential. Information that could be used to identify individuals will not be used in the study report. I am the only person who will know who has taken part. The data will be stored at the Wuthering Heights Hospital and remain confidential.

The results of the project will be printed in nursing and medical journals. There will be nothing in these that could identify anyone who has been part of the study. There is no risk involved in being part of the research.

If you choose not to be part of the study, it will not affect your care. If you decide to take part, and then change your mind, you can choose to no longer participate any time you wish. If you want any information about the project and its results I can be contacted at any time at the above address.

If you have any complaints about the way in which this research project has been, or is being conducted, please, in the first instance, discuss them with me. If the problems are not resolved, or you wish to comment in any other way, please contact the Wuthering Heights Hospital Ethics Committee at the address on this letter.

I will ask you to sign a consent form before we begin.

Thank you for considering my request.

Mary Smith, PhD
1 April 2006

**Figure 2.1** *A sample information sheet.*

## Check List: Items to include in an information sheet

☑ Invitation to participate
☑ An explanation of the project
☑ Implications for their treatment in the health service
☑ Participation is voluntary
☑ Nothing will happen to disadvantage them if they decide not to take part
☑ Any payments or compensation
☑ Who to contact if they want further information
☑ The name and contact details of the principal investigator
☑ The contact details of the ethics committee secretariat

A sample consent form is shown in Figure 2.2, and contains similar facts to the information sheets, but is worded to show that the person agrees to participate, and has a place for them to sign. Some HRECs require a witness to attest to the signing of the consent form, but this is contentious and can be difficult to implement. Check with the ethics committee secretariat to clarify this if you are not sure.

### 'Vulnerable' participants

Some of the most important research that clinical staff can do is with 'vulnerable' participants (children, pregnant women, foetuses, prisoners and the mentally ill). If you are including such people in your study, you need to explain why and what the benefits and safeguards for that population will be. Protecting the participants takes place over the expected benefits of the knowledge that you may generate.

If your subjects are from a vulnerable group who cannot give permission for themselves, and they are too old to gain consent from a parent, for example, mentally ill people with an acute illness episode, then you must gain consent from the relevant advocate. Many countries have systems where the government appoints a 'legal friend' for such people to guarantee their legal rights when they are unable to do so themselves. Find out about this system and how to access it before your research begins. When one is using vulnerable subjects for studies in which there is a degree of risk, and where that risk may be exacerbated by the fact that the subjects are vulnerable – for example, a drug trial for children with cancer – careful planning and a sound understanding of the specific group is required.

Part 1

This consent form is an example of how they can be written; however, some countries have set forms that are mandatory. In the United Kingdom, for example, a standard form is to be used across the country. This can be found at http://www.corec.org.uk/applicants/help/docs/Info_sheet_and_consent_form_guidance.pdf (refer Figure 2.1 and Checklist page 31)

---

**WUTHERING HEIGHTS HOSPITAL
DINGO STREET, LONDON**

## Consent Form

In signing this document, I am giving consent to be part of a study to be conducted by Dr. Mary Smith, from the Wuthering Heights Hospital. I understand that I will be part of a research study to analyse wound care in hospitals. This study will provide guidance for health professionals about appropriate ways to care for patients with wounds.

I understand that I will be asked to participate in a discussion about wound care, which will be taped. The discussion will take about 30 minutes.

My participation was granted freely. I have been informed that participation is entirely voluntary, that even after we begin I can refuse to answer any questions, and can end the interview at any point. I have been told that my answers will not be given to anyone else, and no reports of this study will identify me in any way. I have also been told that my participation (or non-participation), or my refusal to answer questions will have no effect on the services that I receive while in hospital, and that no member of the hospital staff will be told of the content of the discussion.

I understand that the results of this research will be given to me if I ask for them, and that Dr Mary Smith, at the above address, is the person to contact if I have any questions about the study, or my rights as a study participant.

Date. . . . . . . . . . . . . . . . . . . . . . .

Respondent's name. . . . . . . . . . . . . . . . . . . . . . . . . . .

      signature. . . . . . . . . . . . . . . . . . . . . . . . . . . . . .

Witness. . . . . . . . . . . . . . . . . . . . . . . . . . . . . . . . . . .

Investigators' signature. . . . . . . . . . . . . . . . . . . . . . . . . .

---

**Figure 2.2**  *A sample consent form.*

---

### Check List: Informed consent summary

☑ Is the participant competent to consent? If not, guardians need to be approached.

☑ Does the participant have the capacity to make a voluntary choice? If not, guardians need to be approached.

☑ Is the provision of information sufficient? Does your information sheet include methods, demands, risks, conveniences and discomfort?

☑ Have the possible outcomes been explained, for example publication of results?

☑ Is participation voluntary? That is, the participants are not coerced through payment or some other means.

☑ Has it been explained to the participant that they can withdraw at any time without penalty?

---

## ▶ Ethical issues for different groups

Particular ethical issues surround discrete vulnerable groups. We consider some of these as follows.

### Children

What is a child? Most countries use the age of 18 as the cut-off point for childhood; in other words, anyone under this age is deemed a child and is said, legally, to require permission of a parent before consenting to interventions such as surgery, or, in our case, participation in research. However, it has been recognized that young people are able to consent long before the age of 18. A legal precedent, known as the 'Gillick case', exists concerning this issue. It found that children less than the legal age, who are able to consider the implications of their actions and take responsibility for them, are said to be 'Gillick competent' (McLean 2002). So how do we decide that a child is Gillick competent? This has important implications if we are doing a research study, as we need the child's consent before involving them. Of course, if the child is small, then the parent (can be natural parent, step-parent, foster parent or legal guardian) is the one to give consent. But if the child is able to reason and can understand the implications behind their involvement (i.e., is Gillick competent) then the parent's consent is not required. This works well for studies of ethically

Part 1

simple topics, for example, a study of dental hygiene in children. But what if the study is investigating abortion in teenage girls? Or, perhaps, HIV testing? Does the parent have the right to know that their child has participated in a research project about this? Or is that invading the privacy of the child? There are no easy answers to such questions. When faced with this thorny problem, it is best to approach the chairperson of the ethics committee through which your project will be submitted and seek their advice.

## People with a mental illness

Most people with a mental illness will be perfectly competent to give informed consent about participation in a research project. Some, because of their illness, may not be able to reason effectively and so are particularly vulnerable when asked to make a decision about participating. Many societies have legal advocates for people who cannot, for any reason, make a rational and reasonable decision about their own welfare, and so the advocate steps in to decide if whatever the person is being asked to do is in their best interests. If an advocate or a 'legal friend' is available, you will have to apply to them for consent for a vulnerable mental health patient to participate in a study. Depending on the country, this role is taken by the person's closest relation, or someone who has been given power of attorney or been made a legal guardian for that person.

## People with cognitive impairment/intellectual disability

Similarly to people suffering from a mental illness, people with any sort of cognitive impairment or intellectual disability are legally vulnerable, and similar procedures for seeking informed consent are required. This group includes those with a learning disability, dementia, Alzheimer's disease or other impairment of the elderly and acquired brain injury.

## Pregnant women

A pregnant woman is considered vulnerable even though she may be extremely fit and well, because she is responsible for two (or more) lives, the baby's (babies') and her own. Pregnancy, while a normal function of being female, has its own psychosocial dimensions. Researchers have to demonstrate that if pregnant women are included, these dimensions and the particular vulnerabilities associated with them are taken into account when obtaining informed consent and when collecting data.

In a study of, say, young women's attitudes to shopping, many of the women who participate may be pregnant, purely because of the age of your sample, and this will make no difference to your study. In your ethics application, state that your sample may include pregnant women because of the age group chosen, however participation will not affect them in any way. If you are studying the effects of prenatal education and your sample is all pregnant women, you must show that your recruitment procedure does not put any pressure on the women related to their pregnancy. Also, you may have to collaborate with the midwife or obstetrician regarding a woman's participation, depending, of course, on the research project.

## Staff within a specific organization

Imagine you are working in a hospital; the nurse in charge of your ward wants you to be part of their research project, but you do not want to participate. Would you say 'no' if you thought that might affect your position as one of the staff? If, in any organization, a research project recruits its own staff members, then special procedures must be put in place to ensure they give their consent without feeling coerced to do so. Approval must be given by the management as it will impinge on staff's time; however, it may be an important ethical consideration of your research to keep a particular individual's participation confidential. Agreement must be reached with management that the data will remain yours and the reporting of data that will be made public will be unidentifiable, collated data. The employer may want as many people as possible to participate in a project, but people need to be assured that if they do not take part, it will have no effect on their employment. All these considerations should be spelt out in the information sheet.

## Deceased persons

Post-mortem examinations and autopsies require the consent of a relative (except in criminal cases). This includes the removal of body parts for diagnostic or scientific reasons. In 1999, an enquiry was set up at Aler Hey Children's Hospital in Liverpool, UK, to investigate retention of children's organs post-mortem without the consent or knowledge of the parents (Redfern *et al.* 2001). Following this major scandal, which received widespread international media attention, requirements for consent from relatives of the dead have been put in place in all major hospitals and research facilities.

Part 1

## Indigenous people

Indigenous peoples around the world, for example Australian Aboriginal people, American Indians, Arctic Inuit, Maori in New Zealand, have been studied for all sorts of reasons since their first contact with Western civilization; in fact, research of these peoples was often a major consequence of colonization. Most of it was done without the consent of the subjects. Fortunately, it is now recognized that such intrusive research is unethical. In many countries with an indigenous population, any research that seeks to study any aspect of their lives must be reviewed under specific guidelines. Ethics committee secretariats will have information about how such guidelines must be met and will advise you about them. If your research involves community groups, some of the respondents may be indigenous people. In this case, as they are not being studied particularly and are not being treated any differently to the non-indigenous people in your sample, then special approval usually is not required.

---

## ⚠ Hot Tip: Finding ethics resources

In Australia, the National Health and Medical Research Council have recently updated their guidelines on the ethical implications of researching indigenous populations in Australia. Called *Values and Ethics – Guidelines for Ethical Conduct in Aboriginal and Torres Strait Islander Health Research*, these can be downloaded from www.nhmrc.gov.au.

Canada has similar requirements (see http://www.pre.ethics.gc.ca/english/links/links.cfm) as does New Zealand (see http://www.hrc.govt.nz/root/Maori%20Health%20Research/Indigenous_Health_Research.html).

---

## Ethical approval for European populations

Most countries in Europe belong to the European Union (EU) which is in the process of developing standard processes for the ethical review of research in any member country (Europa 2005). In the future, all research ethics application in these countries will be the same, with the same forms and procedures. However, this may take a long time to implement as some of the new countries in the EU (called the 'accession countries') are still developing, and so are their processes for ethical review of research.

Some European countries, for example the United Kingdom, have complicated and lengthy processes for ethical approval of research. These processes, at least for health research, are now centralized through a body called the Council of Research Ethics Committee (COREC). Their website has all the information required, and is at http://www.corec.ac.uk (National Patient Safety Agency 2006).

A word of warning: this website is not particularly 'user friendly' and the application process is lengthy and complicated. Anyone who is contemplating doing any research in the United Kingdom and who has not used the COREC system before would be well advised to seek help from someone who has. This is equally important for all ethics committees and the best place to start to gather accurate information is the research secretariat of the organization with whom you hope to do research and/or the chairperson of the HREC.

▶ **Ethical issues with respect to hearing/observing unethical behaviour**

In undertaking research in a village inhabited by a socially disadvantaged group of people the main subjects were the grandmothers of the family groups. A trusting and ethical relationship with these women was a necessary, yet time-consuming process prior to data collection. One morning, the researcher while having a cup of tea with one of the grandmothers noticed the three-year-old grandson was trying to attract her attention. Grandma was busy talking to the researcher and, after several attempts at shooing the little boy away, she handed the toddler her lit cigarette and the little fellow ran away smoking it. This places the researcher in a difficult situation. If the grandmother was berated for teaching the child to smoke, not only would trust be lost instantly, but many boundaries would have been crossed. This would have made the research, and its promise of privacy and respect, unethical. Not acting on the situation would have been acting unethically as it is not in a three-year-old child's best interests to smoke. Fortunately, the baby health clinic nurse was a well-known and respected member of the community, so, in this situation she was able to be informed. She appropriately cared for the child and family without ever revealing knowledge about the incident. Ethical issues such as these are fairly common in research dealing with communities. While there are no hard and fast rules, it is important to remember that the role of researcher is different to that of clinician, that the trust component of research means one often cannot reveal information that is given in confidence, and that being a researcher can sometimes put

Part 1

one in a compromising position. If you are ever troubled by such a situation, seek the advice of your ethics committee chairperson, or of a senior researcher.

## ▶ Ensuring privacy and confidentiality

Confidentiality is an important ethical consideration. Explain whether the research will involve the collection or disclosure of personal information, for example, from medical records, which may involve a breach of confidentiality. If confidentiality will not be breached because the data to be collected does not include information that would identify individuals, or if the consent of individuals to release the information will be obtained, then discuss this.

Describe the specific steps to be taken to protect confidentiality of data. If data with identifying information will be accessed, specify the person(s) or agency to whom this information will be released. Beware of stating that your study or subjects will be anonymous if they are not. If you collect interview data, then you, or a person on your behalf, will see, or at least hear, the person being interviewed and will know who they are. Interviews can only be anonymous if they are done, for example, over the telephone with the interviewer having no way of identifying the interviewee. Studies where people return questionnaires via unidentified postal envelopes can be anonymous, but if they are returned via email with the respondent's name, or are collected by someone, then they cannot be anonymous. The most such studies can be is 'confidential'.

Anonymity is a difficult term to use in relation to research ethics. While it is usually possible to guarantee confidentiality, anonymity can be more difficult. A project where someone is being interviewed cannot be anonymous as the interviewer sees the interviewee. If the interview is done over the telephone and the phone numbers are unknown then the interview could be anonymous. Coding of questionnaires and interview tools may remove the person's name, however, if a consent form is signed, then even with coding, the project is never truly anonymous. When completing an ethics application, it is important to differentiate between anonymity and confidentiality, and never guarantee anonymity unless you are certain that this is what you have. It is often best to say that you can assure that the data will be kept confidential.

## ▶ Debriefing

There are two aspects of this that are important. First, it is unethical to conduct research without making provision for feedback both to the subjects, and to others involved, for example, staff in a hospital ward who asked their patients if they want to participate in your research.

It is ethical to ask people if they want to be informed of the outcomes of the study in which they are participating. There are many ways of doing this; for example, by taking their postal address and sending them a copy of the report and papers published. Make sure they understand that such processes can take years to happen; for example, some journals might take two years to publish papers which have been submitted. If your study is ongoing over a long period of time, you could send serial 'newsletters' to tell people how it is progressing.

Secondly, provision needs to be made to ensure that if anyone is psychologically or emotionally disturbed by participating in your study, then you have effective procedures in place to help them.

If there is a possibility that people will be disturbed or damaged in any way by participating, explain how you will deal with this. It might be necessary to brief the occupational health nurse in your facility, or perhaps a clinical psychologist, and state in your application that these people will be available should such an event occur.

## ▶ Summary

Unfortunately, the unethical conduct of research has had a long history. In this chapter we have sought to show you how to identify systematically all of the possible ethical implications of your research. If you are at all unsure about any of the ethical implications of your research then take the time to contact your local research ethics committee chairperson and discuss the research with them. If you do not have a committee then use this chapter to consider carefully the ethical implications of your research. In the next chapter we further explore ethical considerations as they pertain to different individual groups and contexts.

Part 1

## ▶ References

Annas, G.J. and Grodin, M.A. (eds) (1992). *The Nazi Doctors and the Nuremberg code: Human Rights in Human Experimentation*. Oxford University Press, New York.

Cave, E. and Holm, S. (2003). Milgram and Tuskegee – paradigm research projects in bioethics. *Health Care Analysis: HCA: Journal of Health Philosophy and Policy*, 11(1): 27–40.

Europa (2005). Research in Europe: ethics committees. Facing the future together. Available from URL: http://europa.eu.int/comm/research/conferences/2005/recs/index_en.htm. Accessed 16 April 2006.

Garrard, E. and Dawson, A. (2005). What is the role of the research ethics committee? Paternalism, inducements, and harm in research ethics. *Journal of Medical Ethics*, 31: 419–23.

McLean, S. (ed.) (2002). *Medical Law and Ethics*. Ashgate, Burlington.

National Patient Safety Agency (2006). Central Office for Research Ethics Committees (COREC). Available from URL: http://www.corec.org.uk/. Accessed 16 April 2006.

Redfern, M., Keeling, J.W. and Powell, E. (2001). The Royal Liverpool Children's Inquiry Report. The House of Commons, London. Available from URL: http://www.rlcinquiry.org.uk/download/chap1.pdf. Accessed 26 February 2007.

Sauerteig, L. (2000). *Ethische Richtlinien, Patientenrechte Und Ärztliches Verhalten Bei Der Arzneimittelerprobung (1892–1931)*. *Medizinhistorisches Journal*, 35(3–4): 303–34.

Shields, L. and Twycross, A. (2003). How research ethics committees work. *Paediatric Nursing*, 15: 36.

# Chapter three

# Multicultural considerations

*Linda Shields*

▶ **Contents**

▷ Doing research overseas
▷ Cultural sensitivity
▷ Disaster and conflict situations
▷ Translations
▷ Research with Indigenous people
▷ Research in developing countries
▷ Politics and research
▷ 'Value adding'

Doing research in a country different to your own can be exciting, is always interesting, and presents a new set of challenges to the researcher. While it may seem obvious to say that all countries are different, it is true. Even when you think the culture of a country may be similar to your own due to shared histories, shared ethnicity and common political systems, because each country has developed individually, and with different pressures, their cultures may be quite dissimilar. A good case in point is Ireland and Australia. Australia's white population consists of many people whose ancestors came from Ireland; both countries are democracies, and most Australians are Christians. Despite what many assume, the cultures in each country are profoundly different, formed by different histories and events. While the Irish engaged in intense political and sometimes violent struggles to free themselves from England, Australians chose to hold ties to Britain. When much of the Irish population migrated to other countries to avoid oppression, Australia took in migrants from many countries, producing a multicultural society. As Australia, with its immense wealth from natural resources, developed one of the world's best health services, Ireland, as the poorest nation in Europe before joining the European Union, has a health service that is still developing. Doing research in different countries means coming to grips with these ideas before one begins. Nevertheless, cross-country and cross-culture research is valuable, interesting and rewarding, not just in research results but in friendships, networks, understanding and tolerance.

Different countries have different ways of doing things, and this, of course, underpins any research planning. Never make the mistake of thinking that because something works one way in one country, systems in another country will be the same. Of course, they may be similar, but always check before you begin.

### ▶ Doing research overseas: cultural considerations

Both within and between countries, different cultures exist. A culture is, 'The totality of socially transmitted behaviour patterns, arts, beliefs, institutions, and all other products of human work and thought' (http://dictionary.reference.com/search?q=culture, accessed 29 April 2006). In some countries, many cultures exist side by side; in others, one culture predominates. Britain and Indonesia both are home to many cultures, while Ireland and Norway have, in the main, one cultural group. All countries will have small populations from other countries. For example, Ireland is home to the Travellers, a small group whose nomadic lifestyle has led to development of a culture different to the predominant Irish. Within each culture there are cultural constructs that guide living and ways of doing things. These include (among others) gender, religion and social class, all of which can influence any research project. A study of the use of medical services by families in countries where female children are valued less than males would have to take gender into consideration. Studies of how spirituality affects health would have to consider different religions, while research about the effect of educational attainment on health would have to include socio-economic status as a factor for examination.

Why do research in countries outside one's own? What use is research in other countries to health professionals working in, say, a charity hospital in America, or a community health clinic in outback Australia? A look at how the Internet has changed communication gives us one reason. The nurse in the charity hospital in the United States can, quickly and easily, find how charity hospitals in other countries work, and find research solutions to problems encountered by nurses there. They may be different to the problems of the nurse in the United States, but they may give the US nurse some ideas about how to do things differently to improve practice.

The nurse in the community clinic in the Australian outback can examine research done by nurses working in, say, remote area clinics in the Canadian north, and see if their ideas can help guide practice in what is, in some ways, a similar situation to that in which the Australian nurse finds himself/herself.

In a wider context, similar research in different countries can build a body of knowledge about specific topics. At present there are several research projects occurring in a range of countries across the world examining the question of whether breastfeeding can protect children and adolescents against obesity (Armstrong and Reilly 2002; Toschke *et al.* 2002; Liese *et al.* 2001; Shields *et al.* 2006a). Results from these projects are beginning to show a trend that this may be the case. While each study is done independently (creating problems of different definitions and different ways of measuring variables), the collective body of work is creating a bank of knowledge about this topic.

Can research in one country be compared with similar research conducted in another country? There are many questions around this, far too many to develop here, however, researchers can set up international studies which can be extremely valuable. The ease of communication provided by electronic media and the ubiquity and ease of air travel have facilitated international research projects, and several funding bodies will give funds for such research. Such projects, especially if well planned and executed, can give wonderful insights into topics under examination. A study of the needs of parents of hospitalized children begun in Iceland now includes Sweden, the United Kingdom, Australia and Indonesia, and negotiations are underway in Iran to conduct the study there (Shields *et al.* 2003; Shields *et al.* 2004; Shields and Kristensson-Hallström 2004; Shields *et al.* 2006b). By using the same questionnaire, slightly modified to take account of differences in language, facilities available in hospitals and parents' expectations of hospital care, interesting results are being revealed which can potentially influence the way children and their families are cared for around the world.

## ▶ Ensuring culturally sensitive research

We have discussed research across countries, with their different cultures, but within countries research can also be conducted across different cultural groups. In fact, any study should take into account the possibility that respondents may come from differing cultural, ethnic or racial groups, as this may have an effect on any findings. Perhaps a researcher may be interested in that very thing – the way different cultures look after their health, for instance. However, caution must be stressed when doing research about the effects of culture on results, and this often has to be taken into account as a confounding variable. For example, a study of the effects of sexual practices on the rate of HIV transmission would have to consider ethnicity as a variable that might confound the results – one ethnic group may consider the use of condoms as perfectly acceptable, while another might think that abstinence from sex the only acceptable way.

Can comparisons be valid? All researchers must think hard about this. Any comparison, for any reason, has to compare like with like, or the comparison is meaningless. A study of the rate of infectious diseases in the United Kingdom will yield a set of diseases different to those in, say, Kenya, and so (apart from showing that they are different) comparisons could not be made between the rates of infectious diseases in the two countries.

### Research in disaster situations

There are two situations in which the rules of cross-cultural research change. In conflict situations, riots, civil unrest, war and natural disasters, researchers have to question the ethics of proceeding with their work. Of course, if the aim of the research is to examine topics related to conflict, war, natural disasters and so on, then the research is, of itself, important. Many of the developments of medicine, for example antibiotics and burns treatments, have come from war. Some of the great advances in health care have come from natural disasters, for example the use of passive exercise to keep paralysed limbs flexible was devised by Sister Elizabeth Kenny during the polio pandemics of the 1930s to 1950s. Research following the Papua New Guinea tsunami in 1998 was used to deal with the effects of the Boxing Day Tsunami in Indonesia in 2004. However, it is wise to question whether it is worthwhile continuing a research project if it is going to put you, the researcher, in any danger. Just as importantly, it may put others at risk as well, for example people with whom you are going to work. Before you leave, refer to your foreign affairs office in your own country to see if there are any travel warnings about the country you are planning to visit. If you are already in the country, register with your own embassy or high commission as someone working on a research visa, so that if any danger does develop, you can be evacuated.

Aid organizations often undertake research in various countries, or support it. There are a range of ethical considerations around such research, especially if the aid recipient is a developing country, or one whose people are particularly vulnerable. A country which fits this situation, and we can use it as an example, is Afghanistan. Any researcher from outside Afghanistan, while supported by an aid agency and there to help the people, would have to be sure that the research they want to conduct really will help the people, rather than just their publication list. This is a rather cynical view, and can be applied to any research conducted in a developing country that is receiving aid from another, but it is an important one nonetheless.

Many countries have large bureaucracies, while others have fewer government controls and offices. Research always comes under bureaucratic scrutiny, and this has to be factored into any proposal for research in a country other than your own. It may take many months and complicated procedures to gain the appropriate government permission to conduct research in some countries, and you may need a specific research visa to do your work there. Always visit the embassy or consulate of the country you wish to visit before you go.

Nursing in some countries is not regarded as a profession with the same status as, say, medicine. To ignore this fact can put your whole project at risk. If you come from a country where nurses and doctors are equal, for example, the Nordic countries, or Australia, you may be offended if you travel to a country where nurses are considered little better than servants, and where you may be treated accordingly. The best tip to prevent this happening is to assess the situation before you go and put in steps to ensure that you have the correct players on your team. It may be critical to make friends with a sympathetic medical doctor, preferably before you go, and have him/her act as your advocate.

## ▶ Trans-cultural research

We have discussed research across cultures, and trans-cultural research is similar, but we use it here to mean research conducted across cultures within a country. There is some debate about the use of the term, and suggestions for others have included 'intercultural' and 'multicultural'. Many countries have different cultural groups living within them, and research projects often examine, for example, the way some aspects of health services are used by different cultural groups within a society, or perhaps expectations of health services by different ethnic populations. In these cases, all the same rules apply as with cross-cultural research, without the considerations of working in foreign country.

Part 1

## Translations

Often, research in another country means translation of questionnaires, interview guides and data, and documents such as consent forms. Accuracy of any translation is vitally important, but becomes even more so when using questionnaires. A question in one language may, on translation to another, mean something entirely different. There is a large literature about translation of research tools, but in the main, the following have to be considered:

---

### ✎ Check List: Translating research materials and findings

☑ Back-translate everything; in other words, once the document has been translated into another language, translate (or have it translated) back into the original language.

☑ Form a panel of experts who use both languages, who can check and recheck your tools.

☑ Check not just translation of words, but translation of concepts; in other words, does something have a different meaning in the target language from the original?

☑ Check questions carefully. Changing questions into other languages can change the direction of the question. A question that might elicit an 'yes' response in English might have 'no' as the usual answer in another language.

☑ Translations can be very expensive. When preparing a grant application, get a full quote from a translation service and include that cost.

☑ Seek the advice of an expert (not just a native speaker) in the other language, preferably someone who is used to translating for research projects.

☑ Test the validity and reliability of the translated questionnaire data once they have been collected in the pilot study and compare the results with the questionnaire in its original language. If the translation is reliable, then the reliability statistics results between the two languages will be similar. Ask a statistician if you do not know how to do this.

---

Most developing countries these days have research ethics committees, so never assume that they do not and begin your research without proper approval. The embassy of the target country will be able to help you with this. If a country does not have research ethics committees, *then make sure you obtain ethical approval from the research ethics committee at your own institution before you leave.* This ensures that you are acting ethically towards the people and the country who will be your hosts and subjects, and will make it easier for papers from the project to be published in reputable journals.

## Working with Indigenous populations

In the past, many countries were colonized by others with scant regard for the original inhabitants. Colonialism reached its zenith in the 19th and early 20th centuries, when many schoolchildren were taught that 'the sun never set on the British Empire'; several European countries governed and exploited others in Asia, Africa and the Pacific regions, and the United States colonized countries such as the Philippines. In all the colonized countries, the original or Indigenous populations were at best governed under a benign oppression, and at worst, were systematically killed to give the land to the new settlers. Independence movements across the world gradually saw colonizing nations either driven out of the colonies, or, in most cases, giving independence to the once colonized. In many countries, though, the settlers from the colonizers stayed, as they had become 'natives' of the country through generations of settlement, while the Indigenous populations, who had by this time become very much in the minority, still suffered from social inequalities and resulting health problems generated by being considered an 'underclass' in the society. Under these circumstances, much research has been done on the Indigenous races of the world. Some of the research has been of immense benefit, bringing with it improvements in health and living conditions. However, much of it has been gratuitous, done for no other reason than curiosity about different ways of life, and conferring no benefit on the subjects. Often it was done with no regard for informed consent or other ethical principles and sometimes resulted in egregious human rights abuses, and offences against cultural beliefs and practices.

This type of poor practice has provoked the need for specific guidelines to be followed and checks and balances put in place to ensure the rights of Indigenous people have been protected. For a research project about Maori in New Zealand, for example, as well as normal ethical approval, researchers must obtain permission from different officials and Maori leaders. This also occurs with Australian Aboriginal people, Canadian Inuit,

Swedish and Finnish Sami people, American Indian populations, and many others. If you cannot find the information you need to do this, ask the ethics committee to whom you are applying for ethical approval to find out for you.

One of the things you may have to do when doing research with Indigenous people is to include someone from that group in your research team. This can become problematic as a fine line can be drawn between real involvement and tokenism. It is insulting to involve someone on the team who cannot understand what the research is about, and so selection of the right person can be tricky. Refer to the leader of the group and seek his/her guidance, make sure they fully understand what you are trying to do, and why you need Indigenous people in your sample. Be sure you outline the benefits for the people, and let them know that you are going to benefit from it too. It would be dishonest to tell them that the benefits are all for them, and they would know that you were not that altruistic. So let them know what is in it for you, as well as for them.

If you plan to pay people, or offer inducements of some kind for people to be involved in your project, check with the leader that this is acceptable. Some societies may be insulted if you offer to pay them for giving assistance; others may be offended if you do not. Do not be scared to ask, better to do so than upset people inadvertently. Research can confer many benefits, so it is quite acceptable to involve Indigenous people as research subjects, however, it must be done with sensitivity and tact.

### Working with Indigenous peoples

The National Health and Medical Research Council of Australia has provided specific guidelines for those researchers that wish to work with Indigenous Australian communities. These can be downloaded from their website at www.nhmrc.gov.au/publications. In New Zealand, Maori people are protected by special legislation that springs from the Treaty of Waitangi that ensures they have control over any research done about them (see http://www.hrc.govt.nz/root/Maori%20Health%20Research/ Indigenous_Health_Research.html). Canada has similar requirements (see http://www.pre.ethics.gc.ca/english/links/links.cfm). Other countries which have Indigenous populations have guidelines for this type of research.

If you decide to work with these communities, you need to be aware of the following values that this group have identified as important in the ethical conduct of research.

> ### Check List: Values relevant to Australian Aboriginal and Torres Strait Islander research
>
> ☑ Reciprocity
> ☑ Respect
> ☑ Equality
> ☑ Survival and protection
> ☑ Responsibility

It is vital when working with these communities that you develop a research question that is important to both parties. This will take time as you sit and work out with communities the best way to proceed. This should be figured into your timeline carefully.

## ▶ Developing country access

We have provided a broad overview of the issues that can be encountered when working in developing countries, however, some warrant special attention. Gaining access to a developing country can be difficult; sometimes research conducted in these countries has been less than ethical, and so governments and people may be wary of researchers who want to come to developing countries. Begin in the embassy or consulate of the country, find out what has to be done, whom best to contact, and what permissions and documents you must have before you can travel there. Always double check this information as it can sometimes happen that the consulate staff may not have encountered applications for entry to conduct research before.

### Permissions

Some countries have bureaucracies and offices set up to deal with people who want to do research in their country, for example, Indonesia requires that all research done by foreigners be registered with *LIPI – Lembaga Ilmu Pengatahuan Indonesia*, the official office of research. Most of these government departments in most countries can be contacted through their websites, and the embassies and consulates of the relevant countries will be able to help you with their processes. However, do not rely on the embassies to let you know about such procedures. You must ask them

Part 1

and insist that they find out the correct procedure for you. In addition, you will often have to go through the local and sometimes national, ethics committees. Government permission will not take the place of ethical review of your research project. If you find that there is no ethics committee available, then ensure it goes through an ethics committee in your home country before you set out. This may be a requirement of overseas countries anyway, and you may end up having to obtain permission from the following ethics committees.

---

### Check List: Ethics approvals for international research

☑ The researchers' local research ethics committee
☑ The national ethics committee of the country you plan to visit
☑ The local ethics committee of that county
☑ The government office that oversees research

---

If your research is about vulnerable or minority groups, you may find that some countries have an extra layer of permission which you must obtain. In Australia, for example, if you want to include Aboriginal people in your study, you must gain permission from the ethics committee in the area in which your project is to take place, plus the special research ethics committee for projects about Indigenous people.

### Bribes

The culture in some countries may work on a system of patronization and payment for favours. Paying a 'fee' for such services can speed up processes such as approval of applications. However, such activities can be construed as bribery and corruption, and must be undertaken with extreme caution. In some places you may find that this is the only way to move your project forward; remember that in many developing countries, people are extremely poor and will try to make money where they can. If you think this might happen, remember to take enough money with you. Nevertheless, it is as well to stay far away from this, and paying 'fees' should only be undertaken as a last resort. Local knowledge and a friend who can help you navigate this minefield are vital.

## Cultural considerations

We could make a long list of things to consider when working in another country, but the best advice is to buy a travel guide to that country – the 'Lonely Planet' series are probably the best – and study the detailed information given about what to do and what not to do in the country you are planning to visit.

## Politics and research findings

Undertaking research in some countries may give rise to rather tricky situations, and it is as well to be aware of these before you begin. You may be given permission to do the research only if your findings can be censored before publication. This can lead to misrepresentation of your results, and if this limitation is put on you, I would advise abandoning the project. Your professional reputation could be jeopardized.

Be sure the government, the heads of the service where your research is taking place, the people with whom you are going to work and your subjects (as appropriate) are aware that you will be publishing your findings in journals, books and so on, which will be open to public scrutiny. If they deny you permission to do so, then you must have a rethink about what you are doing. Some compromise should be sought, but you must never go ahead unless everyone understands your situation.

In a country other than your own (although this will apply to your own country as well) be wary when talking to the media. If your organization has a public relations or media office, seek their help. Do not leave yourself wide open to media scrutiny if you have not done it before, and if you think your research could be misrepresented and misinterpreted. This is particularly important in countries where you are a guest. Offence can derive from the simplest of statements, and it is often wisest to decline to be involved with the media unless you are very sure of yourself and your ability to deal with them.

## Value adding with research findings

Bob Geldof's injunction to 'make poverty history' can be aided by doing research in developing countries. Research is a valuable tool to determine if, for instance, the children in a country would benefit from a research project about diarrhoeal diseases and clean water. Research confers less obvious benefits. Those with whom you work can learn from you as a researcher, and can gain status and perhaps career advancement from being involved in your research project. Remember, though, that you will learn just as much as they will. It is vitally important that you never think that you are going to teach them just because their country is poorer than your own. The people who work in developing countries, especially in health care, all have the same intent towards the people for whom they care, that is, to provide the best and most ethical health care they are capable of providing. This, of course, is the driving force behind anyone who chooses to enter nursing, medicine and the allied health professions in any country, rich or poor. But remember that health professionals in developing countries do this in situations that are far more difficult than their counterparts in the richer nations. This is equally relevant for research. Ethically, any researcher should give something back to the community in which their research is being conducted. This can be done by, say, giving lectures, running seminars, setting up exchanges with one's own country and so on – the list is very long. Look for imaginative ways to do this which will support and add to the host country, but which will not impose any hardship on those participating.

Research findings can greatly improve the health of people, their way of life and their health services. Make sure you publish your findings. It is highly unethical to do research but not to publish the results.

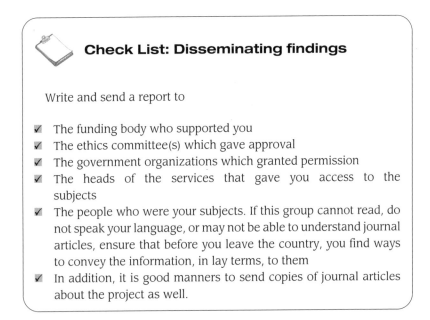

### Check List: Disseminating findings

Write and send a report to

- ☑ The funding body who supported you
- ☑ The ethics committee(s) which gave approval
- ☑ The government organizations which granted permission
- ☑ The heads of the services that gave you access to the subjects
- ☑ The people who were your subjects. If this group cannot read, do not speak your language, or may not be able to understand journal articles, ensure that before you leave the country, you find ways to convey the information, in lay terms, to them
- ☑ In addition, it is good manners to send copies of journal articles about the project as well.

## ▶ Summary

Research with a range of people from different cultures is interesting and exciting, but has to be done carefully, as it is easy to get things wrong, and at best offend, or at worst, make a major error in conducting your research. Homework done before you leave your own country is the best way to prevent problems occurring, and this can take many months to get right. Situations where disaster or conflict has occurred (or is occurring) can yield research which will assist many in the future, but by its very nature, such research involves risk. Assess the situation before you leave your own country and be guided by embassies and travel guidance. Language is a challenge in any research, even in one's own. If you don't ask the right questions the right way, then you won't get the answers you seek. If translation into another language is necessary, there are many techniques to ensure that the translations are correct and culturally relevant.

Undertaking research with Indigenous populations requires extra work to gain access and permission to conduct the research, and also to gain ethical approval. Most countries which have Indigenous people have government bodies from which special approval and permission have to be sought. Different cultures have different ways of doing things, and this is just as relevant for research as for any other aspect of life. It can be very rewarding, and is a great way to gain an understanding of other people and countries.

## ▶ References

Armstrong, J., Reilly, J.J., Child Health Information Team. (2002). Breast-feeding and lowering the risk of childhood obesity. *Lancet*, 359: 2003–4.

Liese, A.D., Hirsch, T., von Mutius, E., Kiel, U., Leupold, W. and Weiland, S.K. (2001). Inverse association of overweight and breastfeeding in 9 to 10-y-old children in Germany. *International Journal of Obesity*, 25: 1644–50.

Shields, L., Hallström, I. and O'Callaghan, M. (2003). An examination of the needs of parents of hospitalised children: comparing parents' and staff's perceptions. *Scandinavian Journal of Caring Sciences*, 17: 176–84.

Shields, L., Hunter, J. and Hall, J. (2004). Parents' and staff's perceptions of parental needs during a child's admission to hospital: an English perspective. *Journal of Child Health Care*, 8(1): 9–33.

Shields, L. and Kristensson-Hallström, I. (2004). We have needs, too: parental needs during a child's hospitalisation. *Online Brazilian Journal of Nursing* (OBJN-ISSN 1676-4285) [online] 2004 December; 3(3). Available in: www.uff.br/nepae/objn303shieldsetal.htm.

Shields, L., O'Callaghan, M., Williams, G., Najman, J. and Bor, W. (2006a). Breastfeeding and obesity at 14 years: a cohort study. *Journal of Paediatrics and Child Health*, 42(5): 289–96.

Shields, L., Young, J. and McCann, D. (2006b). The needs of parents of hospitalised children in Australia. *Journal of Child Health Care*, in press.

Toschke, A.M., Vignerova, J., Lhotska, L., Osancova, K., Koletzko, B. and von Kries, R. (2002). Overweight and obesity in 6- to 14-year-old Czech children in 1991: protective effect of breastfeeding. *Journal of Pediatrics*, 141: 764–9.

# Part two
# Design and implementation of research

# Chapter four

# Writing the 'master' research proposal: gaining ethics approval and funding

*Linda Shields and Sarah Winch*

## ▶ Contents

- ▷ Writing the master research proposal
- ▷ The master research proposal
- ▷ The ethics approval process
- ▷ Using your master research proposal to gain funding
- ▷ Writing a funding application
- ▷ Processes to be established upon receipt of a successful research grant
- ▷ Legal issues and research governance

Of key importance to the success of any research is writing the research proposal. You will be asked to provide this information in many forms over the course of your project. In this chapter we show you how to write a 'master' research proposal that can be used in a number of ways to gain ethics approval, seek funding or be modified into a short form for gaining acceptance for your project. We also explore how to get funding, the process of gaining ethics approval and legal issues associated with the research.

## ▶ Writing the *'master proposal'*

Most ethics, research and funding proposals ask for similar information. By using the following template created by Professor Linda Shields, you can create a 'master' research proposal that addresses ethical and research issues. By addressing all of the criteria, you will find that you have all the requirements necessary to obtain ethics approval and complete funding applications. In addition, summary versions of the proposal make great communication tools when trying to build your team and communicate with staff.

Part 2

Depending on whether you are seeking ethics permission, funding, or access to a designated site, there will be different forms, and formats such as paper or electronic submission. From your *master proposal* you can 'cut and paste' as required onto the various forms that you will need to complete.

## ▶ Template of the master research proposal

### Application data

- Names and addresses, and affiliations of the researchers.
- Provide telephone numbers and email addresses for ease of contact.
- The Principal Investigator (PI) is usually the person leading the research project. Work out ahead of time who is going to be the PI, and who are 'co-investigators'. By negotiating this to everyone's satisfaction before the study begins removes a potential source of conflict later on. Be sure the PI knows that he/she is the person of first contact for the project.
- If it is a student project, for example PhD, then include your supervisor here.
- Length of time the project will take. (A rule of thumb is to work out a time frame and then multiply it by three). Many things can go awry during a research project so a broad time frame is better than a short one.
- This section might ask you about any monies or funding that you already have for the project.
- There might be a space for your signature (or it may be further on in the application forms). If you are submitting the application electronically, you may not need to sign or you may need to organize an electronic signature.

### Purpose and significance of the study

- Explain why you are doing the study.
- Describe what benefit it will bring to the world, profession, people and so on.
- Use simple language, free of technical terms.

### Background

- The literature review goes here.
- Describe what research exists around your topic and provide information about what has been done before. You also need

to provide all the supporting information for your study; for example, the impetus for the research may be a change in policy.

* Include a critical evaluation of existing knowledge, and specifically identify the gaps that the project is intended to fill.
* Explain why you need to do the research.
* Include the research question(s) and/or hypothesis(es).

## Characteristics of the subject population

* What is the age range of participants? For example, you might say that all the subjects in your study about the health of a group of working men are aged between 18 and 65 years.
* What is the gender of the participants? If you have more of one group than another, explain why, for example, a study of nurses will probably have more women than men because it is a female-dominated profession. Equal opportunity legislation in some countries will require you to include equal numbers of both sexes. If your study is specifically about one group, explain it. An example could be a study of prostate cancer. You would include a sentence such as 'only men are to be included in this study because only males contract prostate cancer'.
* Inclusion criteria: who you are including and why? For example, in a study of childbirth amongst a poor population of a big city you would say that to be chosen in the study, subjects would have to be on government welfare, be in the last trimester of pregnancy, and be single mothers.
* Exclusion criteria: who you are excluding and why? For example, in the study of the childbirth experiences of poor women, you might say that you are excluding black women because they have different cultural practices to your included group and these might influence findings if you include them. However, if you are excluding minority groups and it could be seen as racist not to include them, you have to state why. This does not mean you always have to include minority groups; you may be studying white Anglo-Saxon men in a place where they are the majority of the population, but you need to state this as a reason for excluding others.

## Method of participant selection

* Describe the way in which potential participants will be identified and recruited. Outline how you are going to recruit

**Check List (Continued)**

subjects. If you are using advertisements, save a copy for the ethics application.

• Explain the processes you are going to use for recruitment. If you are going to recruit by using an information sheet for potential participants to read, and then re-contact them to see if they would like to participate, explain this.

• If you are planning to pay people to participate, discuss this here.

• If you plan to give participants gifts instead of payment, explain.

• Develop and attach a participant information sheet and consent form. See Figures 2.1 and 2.2

## Study site

• State the location(s) where the study will be conducted.

• If your subjects are to be drawn from a variety of sites, list them.

• If this is the case, you may have to submit HREC applications to each of them. Once you have ethical approval, state this also and attach a copy of the approval letter.

## Methods and procedures applied to human participants

• Describe the study design and all procedures to be applied.

• Discuss if it is a quantitative or a qualitative study, a randomized trial, a survey, a phenomenological study; in other words, describe the research methods, what you are going to do and how you are going to do it.

• If you are doing a drug trial, attach the drug protocol; if you are using questionnaires or interview plans, attach them.

## Sample size

• For a qualitative study describe how many subjects you plan to include.

• For a quantitative study explain the way in which the sample size was calculated, and provide justification of the sample size in terms of its statistical validity. You should include your power calculation that will tell you whether your sample has the power it needs to provide the answer you need. It is good idea to consult a statistician about this.

## Data analysis

- Provide details of the data analysis techniques to be used.
- If you plan to determine which tests to use after the data has been collected, so that you can conduct the most appropriate test according to what the data looks like, say so. However, if this is the case, you will have to justify this quite strongly as ethics committee members and funding bodies will want to know whether you have some idea of what you are doing as opposed to collecting data without any real idea of how you are going to deal with it.

## Primary and secondary outcomes

- Identify your endpoint. This should be an outcome of some kind.
- Provide details on how outcomes are going to be measured, for example, if parents' needs are being investigated in a study using a questionnaire, you may measure how well they communicate with staff. Your primary outcomes from this might be improved communication between parents and staff, and secondary outcomes will be improved care for the families.
- Explain how you will measure outcomes.
- Outcomes may also include papers submitted to peer-reviewed journals, a report for the institutions in which the research took place and for the ethics committee.

## Potential benefits and risks

- List the good things that will come from your study.
- Describe the potential benefits of the study in terms of human health/welfare, the advancement of knowledge or the good of society.
- List potential risks/discomforts/inconveniences. A risk is a potential harm associated with the research to which a reasonable person in the participant's position, if warned of the risks, would be likely to attach significance. Risks can be physical, psychological, sociological, economic and legal; for example, if your study requires blood samples, you would have to explain that some pain might occur. For trials of treatments where data already exists, it might be possible to calculate statistically the chances of an unwanted side effect occurring, for example, in a trial of a new wound dressing, previous data might be able to be used to show that in 200 subjects, there is a 1% chance of necrosis of good tissue when the treatment is used; in other

**Check List (Continued)**

words, if data are available, you can estimate the probability that a given harm may occur. Discuss how this will be handled and any potential reversibility of any ill effect.

## Risk classification, protection and risk benefit relationship

- Classify your risks as less than minimal, minimal, greater than minimal, life threatening. Estimating levels of risk can be easy, for example, if one is testing a new cyto-toxic treatment for cancer, then it may carry obvious life-threatening risks to the people on whom it is being trialled, and this would be called 'life-threatening level of risk'. At the other end of the spectrum, if one were studying the effectiveness of a healthy lifestyle programme, then it would carry a less than minimal risk to the subjects.
- Describe the procedures you will use to minimize and/or manage the potential risks identified previously.
- Explain here how the risks associated with your research are outweighed by the good the results might bring about; for example, you might say that while there is a 1% chance of tissue necrosis with the new wound dressing under trial, there is a probability that it will benefit 80% of the people in the trial.
- If no special indemnity arrangements need be made for research participants, indicate this and explain why.
- Many institutions will have prescribed indemnity arrangements to which you will have to adhere, and this can be discussed with managers and heads of departments when you meet with them. Attach any forms/letters relating to this.

## Therapeutic alternatives

- Some HRECs will want you to explain (if relevant to your study) what therapeutic alternatives are available to subjects outside of a research study; for example, in a study of wound care treatment, you could describe alternative dressings available to subjects.

## Budget and budget justification

- Write the budget for the project.
- Provide a breakdown of the way in which funds will be spent according to set categories. These are usually personnel,

infrastructure, equipment, maintenance costs, travel and accommodation.

- If your study requires the services of a pathology, pharmacy or radiology department, written confirmation from the Director of Pathology, Director of Pharmacy and/or the Director of Radiology (or equivalent) that the resource implications have been considered and funds are available to cover the costs will be required.
- Research that affects the workload of staff of a facility or service should have an approval letter from the relevant Head of Department/Division and/or the Director or equivalent. By this stage we expect that this person has been informed and has given approval for the study to proceed.
- Local nursing staff are excellent for accessing potential participants, gaining their consent and collecting data. These processes can be time-consuming, therefore, personnel such as these need to be well resourced within the budget.
- Any payment or inducement to participate in the research must be described. Also, outline the financial obligations that the participant will incur as a result of participating in the study, for example subjects might have to pay bus fares to travel to where the research is being carried out.
- Explain if the participant will incur costs over and above what would normally be incurred by standard treatment, for example additional diagnostic/follow-up tests, longer hospitalization. Provide details of these. If no additional costs will be incurred, then say so. Describe economic incentives or other rewards for participation, and procedures that must be completed by participants in order to receive either full or partial compensation. If participants will not receive compensation for participation, explain why not.
- Be sure to add up all your expenses carefully. *Get this checked!* Incorrect addition on budgets is one of the most common errors in a grant proposal.
- You need to include all of the reasons why you have requested your funds in the way that you have in the budget justification section.

## Timelines

- Identify all the milestones for your project and write a timeline against these.
- A 'Gantt' chart can be useful in planning your project against a timeline

Part 2

**Check List (Continued)**

## Approval letters and potential assessors

- Attach signed approvals from your line manager and/or the manager in the service/facility/institution in which your study will be conducted.
- If it is a multi-site study, you will most likely need signatures from each site.
- If your study is being funded by a granting body, drug company or from any source whatsoever, attach this information as well. This can pose problems, particularly if funding comes from a commercial source, for example a drug company, so you may need to discuss this with the HREC chairperson.
- Some funding applications will ask you to nominate assessors for your project. This allows you to nominate an expert who you know will be able to make an informed assessment of your project. At this point start thinking about whom you will use. It is vital that you ask permission of the person you nominate before you include their names on any grant application. It is possible, also, to name people who you do not want to review your application. By providing the names of people who you know have a stake in not wanting your research to go ahead, or who may be obstructive for any reason, alleviates the possibility of embarrassment for all. If you are unsure then leave this section on the grant application blank.

## Information sheets and consent forms for participants

- Write in plain language suitable for your potential participants.
- Explain the purpose of the study and what is going to happen.
- Clearly state what is required of the participant.
- List the benefits and risks.
- Carefully explain any remuneration.
- Information and consent sheets should be separate.
- Leave space on each document for the three signatures required: participant, researcher and witness.

## Disseminating findings

- Say how you will disseminate your findings. Usually this will be through poster presentations, reports and refereed journals.

## ▶ The ethics approval process

### Deciding to obtain ethical approval

Once you have developed your *master proposal*, you need to decide whether you need to obtain ethics approval. This can be confusing; especially in countries with highly bureaucratized systems of government and health care in which audits of performance are commonplace. For example: Is the systematic reporting infection rates following surgery research or audit? Do surveys of patient satisfaction constitute research? Retrospective chart audits are often used to examine how effective a specific treatment might be. Is this audit or research? This thorny question generates much debate, and governments and 'watch dog' bodies have produced many documents in an attempt to answer the question.

The implications for HRECs are wide ranging, as ethical approval is required for research, but not for audit. Some people may be tempted to declare their research as audit to try to avoid having to apply for ethical approval. If the project is, in reality, a research study, then this is unethical practice. Consider the matters raised in Chapter 2. Do any of these apply to your project or the project you are being asked to support? Generally, we seek ethical approval because we need to protect research subjects from unethical practice and the researcher and the institution from the consequences of such action.

---

### Check List: Deciding to get ethical approval

- ☑ The project compares procedures that are not in common use with other procedures that are established and considered 'normal'.
- ☑ The study accesses personal information for purposes other than finding out about things like patient satisfaction, or the counting or measuring factors such as infection rates, or length of stay, and so on.
- ☑ The project will increase knowledge in your discipline, and uses questionnaires, interviews and so on; or uses human tissue or organs (from either the living or dead), or that collected for other reasons, such as clinical examination.
- ☑ The study uses observation of, for example, behaviours, or actions, or the study of physiological effects of the body.
- ☑ Clinical trials of drugs and treatments.
- ☑ The project involves radiation, X-rays or other imaging techniques.

Part 2

**Check List (Continued)**

☑ The study involves some sort of surgical procedure, no matter how minor.
☑ The project examines a new or innovative practice.
☑ The study involves video or audio taping participants.
☑ The project is covert. This means that participants do not know that they are being observed. This type of study method is used frequently when observing hand washing (or lack thereof) amongst healthcare professionals.

If you are unsure whether your project requires ethical approval, ask the secretary of your local ethics committee. It is better to enquire first than have your study suspended or stopped because you did not obtain ethical approval before you started.

## ! Hot Tip: Resources to assist with ethics applications

**Australian resources:**
National Health and Medical Research Council
See www.nhmrc.gov. au/publications

1. National Statement on Ethical Conduct in Research Involving Humans
2. Guidelines for Ethical Conduct in Aboriginal and Torres Strait Islander Health Research

**UK resources:**
The Central Office for Research Ethics Committees (COREC)
www. corec.org.uk
Ethics Research Information Catalogue (ERIC) www.eric-on-line.co.uk

### Feedback from ethics committees

If your application needs clarification, some committees will invite you to attend a meeting and explain your project. They will ask you to clarify points in the project which they do not understand fully before they give approval. Once you have submitted your application, one of three things will happen.

1. You will be given approval immediately.
2. Your application will be rejected.
3. You will receive a letter or email asking for clarification of aspects of your application which you will have to answer before approval will be given.

For most researchers scenario 3 is the most common. Few people have their projects approved immediately, and very few projects are rejected out of hand. Do not be discouraged if you are asked to review and explain parts of your application. It is important for all involved that your study meets the highest ethical standards, and HRECs are there to assist you to do this!

## ! Hot Tip: Ethical approval is vital

It is completely unacceptable to go ahead with a study without some sort of ethical review. Journals will rarely publish a paper unless ethical review has been given to the study it describes, and you must note that you had approval when you write the paper. For more information about ethical research, see Chapter 2.

## ▶ Using your master research proposal to gain funding

Research is a labour-intensive exercise and is unlikely to proceed on the good will and motivation of the persons involved. Part of conducting research is securing adequate funding. Many different types of grants exist and you may draw on a variety to complete a project. In one example we know of, a group of emergency nurses wanted to study the effects of resuscitation of critically ill patients on their families. It was a small study (Holzhauser *et al.* 2006) that managed to gain a total of AUD 8274 sourced from a hospital charitable foundation, a local nurses association and an equipment company.

To start your search, first check what is available through your healthcare facility or academic organization. Offices of research, located in universities, compile and promote a calendar of grants that are available for researchers. Some of these grants are discipline-specific such as in the area of diabetes or asthma. Other grants are based on the profile of the applicant or the form and/or nature of the research project.

**Part 2**

> ### Check List: To help locate research funding sources
>
> ☑ Facility research and quality budgets. These are great for small amounts of funding to start a project.
> ☑ Facility research charities and foundations.
> ☑ Peak interest bodies for specific diseases, such as the Asthma Society, The Cancer Fund.
> ☑ Facility and/or University Offices of Research.
> ☑ Electronic Research Bulletin boards from government or industry.

## Types of grants

There are many different types of grants available that suit researchers at different stages of their career as the following list demonstrates. Some require substantial track records and who you have on your team will help in these cases. However, many finding bodies including governments are committed to assisting the next generation of researchers to begin their careers.

### Early career researcher grants

These are great for those at the start of their career as they do not require the researcher to have a strong track record. Instead they provide researchers early in their career with an opportunity to gain experience in grant applications, research methodology, project implementation and reporting procedures.

### New staff grants

These are available at some of the larger, research intensive health facilities, when staff move into research positions. If you have been asked to accept a research portfolio or position, you should ask whether there is a 'start up' grant attached to the role. You may be surprised at what is available!

### Project grants

Designed to provide funding support for quality research projects with modest financial costs, these are often small grants. Nevertheless, they provide an excellent opportunity to kick start a pilot study that may lay the foundation for further work.

### Implementation and service evaluation grants

Gaining popularity in the health sector, these grants involve identifying a practice problem, implementing research evidence and evaluating the outcome.

*Collaborative research grants*
Designed to foster collaborative research between organizations such as a hospital and a university, these grants are especially popular in Australia as part of the Australian Research Council's linkage scheme.

*Program grants*
These are large-scale grants that will fund a program of research over a number of years. They are often directed towards the bioscience community as they have significant costs in establishing laboratories and generally require the research team to have a well established track record.

---

## ! Hot Tip: Finding a grant reader

Applying for a grant is highly competitive. This means that not all grants are funded and you may miss out. Your research proposal needs to be developed to a high standard. Having access to a grant readership scheme is particularly useful for beginning researchers. This means that when you have finished writing your grant (drawn from your *master proposal*), it is circulated for reading and feedback from more experienced researchers. Most universities offer this service for researchers. If you work in a healthcare facility then ask a more experienced researcher to look at your grant.

---

You will also need to demonstrate that your team has the capacity to deliver the research outcomes, that is, completion of previous research projects through to publication. This is known as 'track record' and is a central criterion for judging the many requests that granting bodies receive for funding. If you do not have the track record then you need to build a team around you that does. We have given hints on how to do this in Chapter 2.

### Writing a funding application
If you type into Google 'writing grant applications', you will get 30,300,000 responses in 0.33 seconds. If you need help writing your application you may decide to consult Google! Alternatively, we suggest that you get some help from the people working on your team who have been successful previously with grant writing and who should know your topic well. In this section we provide some broad guidance on managing the funding application process.

**Part 2**

Funding guidelines usually contain the eligibility criteria, the desired format for the research proposal, timelines, what can be included and what is to be excluded in the budget. Some will also contain how proposals are to be evaluated. Refer to your Master Research proposal! If you have followed the template then you will have, if not all, most of the information you need. Use your *master proposal* to cut and paste what you need into the application. Address all aspects of the application carefully. You will often find that you are not given much space to write about your project, so you will need to develop a clear and concise style. Again a grant reader can help you with this.

## ! Hot Tip: Follow the guidelines precisely

You need to obtain the guidelines and follow them to the letter! If there is something that you do not understand – request clarification. This is particularly important if you are not sure whether you are eligible to apply for the grant. Once you have completed the application, go through it very carefully and ensure all sections are complete, and all attachments included. Make sure that you provide exactly what the requesting body asks for. That is, if the funding body or ethical guidelines request '20 copies' then provide 20 copies. If you do not follow their instructions with the utmost care, your application may be excluded or held over to the next meeting.

In order to maximize your funding opportunities spend some time finding out about the organization that you are approaching. Request a list of funded projects, and an annual report from the selected funding body. This will give you an idea of what they are funding and what directions they will take in the future.

The following checklist will also give you some guidance.

## Check List: Maximizing funding opportunities

☑ Check to see that the research funding will meet your project's budgetary needs.
☑ Identify the relevant funding conditions in relation to the timing of ethics clearances. Funding may be jeopardized if clearance is not obtained within a specified date.

☑ Make sure you allow time for all the signatures required. Many forms require that the 'head of the institution' sign the form. By the nature of their position these people are often very busy and you will need time (sometimes up to one week) to get their signatures.

*Other budget considerations*

When developing the budget, all resource implications have to be identified so that the budget accurately reflects the project costs. Do not be tempted to 'skimp', that is, make the research look inexpensive in order to secure funds as this will eventually place too much of a burden on the team members and/or alternatively compromise the integrity of the work. Conversely, do not try and claim for unwarranted time and resources, such as computers and software that you want to keep after the project. Funding bodies are adept at recognizing a 'padded' budget.

**Maximizing 'in-kind support'**

Most funding bodies look for evidence that the institution that is conducting the research supports the project and is willing to make some contribution. This is often recognized through the provision of in-kind support. Most healthcare facilities are able to muster a small amount of in-kind support such as office space, parking, staff release time or library access. If your team involves an academic staff member then basic research support such as library services should be available through their institution. The following checklist details the variety of in-kind support that can be useful when forming your application.

### Check List: Kinds of 'in-kind support'

☑ Access to computing systems
☑ Access to library facilities
☑ Access to networked information retrieval facilities
☑ Physical accommodation, office, 'hot' desk, computer
☑ All risks insurance and professional indemnity insurance
☑ Animal and human ethics clearances
☑ Safety clearances
☑ Financial management and auditing

Part 2

**Check List (Continued)**

☑ Secretarial and administrative support
☑ Basic services such as power and telephones
☑ Staff release time
☑ Parking
☑ Meeting rooms
☑ Travel vouchers

## Submitting grants

Whether the submission is being prepared for consideration of funding or ethics approval, it is wise to identify the date well in advance and plan accordingly. If you are uncertain about anything in the application form, it is always a good idea to contact the nominated person usually identified in the information guide. It is far better to sort out anything that may be confusing before you submit the application.

## Getting help with funding applications

If you have a research office based at your facility, they can provide you with current guidelines and application forms for external granting bodies. Research office staff can also advise you on completing the necessary forms and may read your application prior to submission. While they are not content experts or even necessarily experienced researchers, they can check that you have provided all the information that is required and eliminate any technical grounds for exclusion. Some offices will also check that the research plan is clear and that you have explained your methodology in enough detail. They can also check the budget to determine if appropriate salaries and on-costs have been used and if any taxes should be included. This takes time so research offices often have a cut-off date for the receipt of funding applications that precedes that of the funder by about 3 weeks. Make sure you include this in your planning.

## Processes to be established upon receipt of a successful research grant

Congratulations! You have been successful in getting some funds to conduct your research. There are some more steps for you to follow in establishing the grant and progressing through the contract phase. If you have a research office at your facility then they can help you with this process. If not, the following checklist will help you record and monitor the grant.

## Check List: Establishing a grant file

You will need to establish a grant file that contains

- ☑ a copy of the successful grant
- ☑ a copy of ethics statements
- ☑ written advice from the granting body offering the funds
- ☑ a copy of any conditions of grant and/or the acceptance form
- ☑ a copy of the details provided to the relevant Faculty Business Manager with a request that a new cost-centre be opened
- ☑ a copy of the research grant contract
- ☑ a copy of all your approval letters

Grant money is very precious and needs to be used for exactly what it is intended, the conduct of research as per your funding application. If you work in a large health care facility, establish a specific cost centre for the research monies. This money needs to be protected until the end of the project and cannot be used for other purposes. Although research contracts may be tiresome, they at least specify in law what can and cannot be done with the awarded funds and therefore offer some protection to researchers working within healthcare facilities where funds may be tight!

## Hot Tip: Keeping financial records of grant money

Keep up-to-date financial records specifically to track how the money has been spent. Keep your evidence of this such as audited financial statements.

### Adhering to an approved research plan/protocol

The application you submit to an ethical or funding body is the proposal that you must adhere to. If you change any aspect of your protocol, you need to advise the ethics committee, funding body and organization who have all consented to the project. If you change your proposal substantially, you need to submit another application. If you do find yourself in the position of having to make changes, consult the secretary of your relevant committee and ask for advice on whether an amendment to protocol will

Part 2

suffice or a new application is required. For funding bodies you usually need to sign a contract that states funding is given for that specific project and purposes only. Funds can potentially be withdrawn if there is a considerable deviation from the study for which funds were granted.

---

## ! Hot Tip: Signing of contracts and agreements – acceptance of grants

As a researcher working in a healthcare facility or a university the responsibility for signing research agreements and contracts rests with the facility. In the case of research contracts, facility staff (often with a legal background) should review the agreement to ensure that the facility's (and researcher's) interests are protected. They may negotiate on behalf of the researcher on areas such as indemnity, ownership of intellectual property rights and protection of the rights of researchers to publish their results.

---

## ▶ Legal issues and research governance

### Ownership and control of data

Generally speaking, data collected by a researcher remain the property of that individual (or group of researchers). In some cases, ownership can be transferred to someone else, for example under specific contractual arrangements with funding bodies, or perhaps health authorities who oversee the facilities from where the data are collected. If there is the slightest suggestion that anything different is occurring, it is important for researchers, particularly if new to research, to seek advice from trusted colleagues, or from a lawyer. This becomes even more important if your research could result in a patent, and from which you stand to make money, for example if you invent something.

If you are involved in research that may produce a commercial benefit (such as a device, process, procedure or computer program), the organization that you work for may also have a claim in any future benefits. They may share the intellectual copyright with you or own it altogether. These issues are complex whether you work in the tertiary sector or a health service, and if you think that your research may fall into this area then you need to seek advice early on from your office of research, the health facilities lawyers or a private legal firm that specializes in intellectual copyright.

## Contracts with service providers and funding bodies

Before the grant money is passed over to you, there is likely to be a contract of some kind to sign. Seek some advice before signing and read the contract well. Most granting bodies will have few restrictions on your research – after all, they would not have given you the money if they did not like your proposal, but you must know what it is you are signing before you begin.

It will probably include clauses about intellectual property rights, access to subjects, how and where you will present your findings and may include a clause about indemnity; in other words, who can be sued if anything goes wrong during the research and a subject is harmed. If you are unsure of what you should be signing then seek advice from a legal officer experienced in this type of work.

## Indemnification

In case adverse events arise from your study, it is important to provide evidence of indemnification for research participants. The trend to sue for compensation for a perceived injury is growing and HRECs are aware of the need to ensure all procedures are in place to protect institutions, services and, most importantly, research subjects and investigators. Of course, in studies with less than minimal risk, this may not be necessary. If you are unsure about your needs in this area then consult the Office of Research if you work in a university or your legal experts if you work in a healthcare facility.

## Research governance

In the United Kingdom, a whole new facet of research ethics approval has developed, mainly in the Department of Health, though it affects research in most disciplines. Commonly known as 'research governance', it sets standards for roles and responsibilities for those who wish to undertake or be involved in research studies. The British guidelines provide a framework for ensuring that roles and responsibilities are well delineated. If you are planning to conduct research in the United Kingdom, then it would be advisable to consult the speciality websites about research governance. The best place to start is with http://www.dh.gov.uk/PolicyAndGuidance/ResearchAndDevelopment/ ResearchAndDevelopmentAZ/ResearchGovernance/fs/en (Department of Health 2005).

**Part 2**

## ▶ Summary

Undertaking research is rarely problem free, but careful planning certainly can go a long way to assisting smooth progress. While time-consuming at first, if you follow the *master proposal* detailed in this chapter, you should have a research document that will be of use for communication purposes, grant applications and ethics approval. Conducting research is not just about creating new knowledge. There are significant areas of risk that both you as the researcher and your organization can be exposed to if you do not meet your legal obligations. In this chapter we have touched on some of these and provided you with links to find out more. It is an area that is becoming increasingly more complex and needs regular review by active researchers.

## ▶ References

Department of Health (2005) Research Governance Framework for Health and Social Care (second edition). Department of Health, London.
Holzhauser, K., Finucane, J. and De Vries, S.M. (2006). Family presence during resuscitation: a randomised controlled trial of the impact of family presence. *Australasian Emergency Nursing Journal*, 8(4): 139–47.

# Chapter five

# Identification, access and recruitment of research subjects

*Amanda Henderson*

'The rubber hits the road'

## ► Contents

▷ Identification and location of the target population
▷ Building bridges to potential participants
▷ Making contact with the population
▷ When timing is crucial
▷ The value and limitations of databases
▷ Planning the amount of time in the field: deliberations and considerations
▷ Maximizing retention: trials and longitudinal studies

Of central importance to the success of any research study is the recruitment of suitable research subjects. To do this, you need to identify appropriate environments to gain access to your target research population. Frequently, these groups are located within healthcare facilities where a significant amount of gate keeping is present both in terms of staff and patient populations. In this chapter we share ways of negotiating this maze so that you can approach and recruit sufficient research subjects to make your project a success.

A key factor in negotiating this maze effectively is keeping people on side. The contacts you make and build upon can be instrumental in maximizing your exposure to the target group. Recruitment of participants often represents the largest single component of the workload

Part 2

in a research project, yet it can often receive the least consideration. Poor attention to detail when locating, accessing and recruiting participants can result in small non-representative samples (Aitken *et al.* 2003). Once you have clearly identified your participant group, you can make arrangements for access. This should be done in conjunction with the time period(s) that will provide the most informative data, to answer the specific question being asked. We explore this further in Chapter 6.

## ▶ Identification and location of the target population

In your *master proposal* you will already have identified key personnel to approach. Hopefully, you will have taken our earlier advice and secured a champion and sponsor and built a team with diverse strengths, including contacts within the target population. Ideally, this includes links to clinicians at the local level (i.e., the unit that you want to recruit either patients or staff!). Once you have secured your ethical approval (*never before*), you need to make arrangements regarding access to research populations.

Ideally, ethics committees ensure that the research team has consulted the Head of the Department (HOD) of the area that is to be accessed. Alternatively, the HOD is part of the research team. In any case, agreement by the department should be gained in writing.

## ⚠ Hot Tip: Agreement about resources

Agree, in writing, to the use (if any) of local resources prior to the commencement of the project, for example, the use of administrative staff to distribute forms or surveys. Also, ensure that the staff are willing to comply with this request. Try and offer something in exchange for assistance with the project.

While the head of department may have agreed to let you recruit from their area, you still need to work with the local staff for access. Ethical clearance does not usually grant 'automatic' access to the population requested in your proposal.

## ! Hot Tip: Determine a strategy whereby your research receives priority attention

Your research tasks constitute just one activity that is occurring in a myriad of many other healthcare practices within the organization you have selected to undertake data collection. Your tasks need to be considered in relation to other priorities and processes integral to the practice area. Depending on how you have framed your research question in terms of how it enhances core business will determine the priority the research receives within busy environments.

---

Before you organize access, clearly identify the participant population. This should be specified in your *master proposal*. You also need to decide when and where these potential participants are best recruited from. This will be informed by your research question and study design. For example, a pre- and post-test design will mean that you need to recruit before and after your intervention.

---

## ! Hot Tip: Ensure you have an adequate budget for recruitment

Don't underestimate the time and difficulty required to recruit participants. Many unexpected situations can arise, for example, consultants take leave during national conferences/seminars and services may be reduced. Alternatively, extraneous personnel, that is, you the researcher, may be excluded from specific clinical areas due to concerns about the spread of infection. It is wise to extend your anticipated recruitment phase and the budget.

---

### ▶ Building bridges to potential participants

In Chapter 1 we explained the importance of developing the correct team. The correct team with a senior champion and local sponsor will ensure a seamless transition between the researchers and all relevant levels of the healthcare facility. You will need all of this expertise to locate your

**Part 2**

target population and facilitate the desired access required for both quant-itative and qualitative research. If you have assembled the correct team, your efforts will now begin to show results. Local knowledge is invaluable in locating, identifying, accessing and recruiting potential populations. Detailed preparatory work with local community and/or health agencies can help you avoid the following that can significantly curtail the size of your data set (of particular concern for quantitative research):

1. Time wasted on accessing populations who do not have participants who 'fit' the criteria of the research project
2. Missed opportunities for recruiting participants because a member of the research team is not present to recruit
3. Incomplete data sets that can not be included in the analysis because insufficient time has been allowed for completion or 'follow-up' data has been lost
4. Exposure of participants in your study to other events, external to your research, that may skew or influence your data.

Unrestricted access to the target population is preferred for quantitative data where reasonable response rates are required. Alternatively, for qual-itative data it is not the response rate but rather the 'quality' of the data collected that is important. In this case local knowledge facilitates the researcher(s) access to participants that are most likely to share narratives and descriptions rich in the content area that is sought.

For example, a researcher exploring the experiences of registered nurses who support student learning in the clinical context was linked (through effective networking) to a clinical area where many students were placed. This meant that nearly all of the staff who were accessed and able to be invited to participate 'fitted' the inclusion criteria (Walker 2006). This assisted in maximizing the researcher's efforts regarding recruitment.

## Making contact with the population: when and how to access populations

Following the identification of your target population, you need to determ-ine when and how you are going to access them. For example, individuals with mental health issues maybe located in the community but may be more easily accessed in a mental health in-patient facility or outpatient clinic. You should also check that your recruitment location will not preju-dice the question that is being asked. For example, for your study accessing mental health patients, you need to determine if there is any bias from recruiting at the outpatient's clinic.

### ► Advertising

Accessing participants from the community or from a facility as a whole requires strategic marketing, including advertising to reach the population group. Advertisements need to be approved by the research ethics committee. In your advertisement you need to include the following:

---

 **Check List: Participant advertisements – content to be included**

☑  Why the research is being conducted
☑  You and your team's credentials
☑  Potential gains for the participant and the broader community
☑  Time commitments for prospective research participants, the anticipated time and duration of interactions with the researcher(s)
☑  The nature of the interaction, for example, an interview, or some form of stress or exercise testing
☑  The proposed location of the data collection, that is, where the research participant would need to travel
☑  Appropriate remuneration for travelling expenses for the participant or whether a gift such as a movie voucher will be given as an appreciation
☑  Potential benefits for the participant other than direct monetary payment or a gift
☑  Your contact details

---

### ⫶ Hot Tip: Displaying advertisements

You will need permission from the Marketing and Communications department or the Chief Executive Officer to display your advertisement in most clinical facilities. Generally, you cannot decide yourself where to put up your poster. There is usually a lot of competition for advertising space in large hospitals and this is where your champion can help!

Part 2

You may also like to advertise in your local newspaper. The following is an example provided courtesy of Ms Letitia Burridge who is conducting a study examining care giver reluctance associated with patients who have cancer.

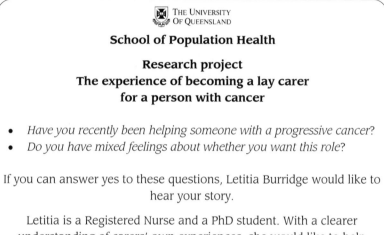

THE UNIVERSITY
OF QUEENSLAND

## School of Population Health

### Research project
### The experience of becoming a lay carer
### for a person with cancer

- *Have you recently been helping someone with a progressive cancer?*
- *Do you have mixed feelings about whether you want this role?*

If you can answer yes to these questions, Letitia Burridge would like to hear your story.

Letitia is a Registered Nurse and a PhD student. With a clearer understanding of carers' own experiences, she would like to help develop better support for carers of people with a cancer.

**For more information, or if you would like to be involved, please phone Letitia on 3365 5556.**

These general advertisements directed at the broader population are variable in the interest that they generate. However, if the advertising is specifically targeted to certain populations, for example, a study designed to 'enhance limb movement in older persons' is specifically advertised within literature or magazines directed at seniors, or displayed on posters in retirement settings, then the interest in the research and hence the number of potential participants can be much higher.

While populations in the community, when clearly articulated and identified, can provide a rich source of clinical data about health in our broader population, access to specific health agencies such as hospitals or long-stay facilities are useful for research into specific groups at designated periods along the continuum of health care. Research drawing on populations across the wider community, often referred to as the 'public', can reveal very different findings to specific populations in healthcare facilities.

## ▶ Entering healthcare facilities

### Who to consult?

In Chapter 1 we show you how to make contact with the people in the organization who can assist you progress your research. If you have not done this thus far then the time has definitely come to make contact! Accessing the requisite population for your project requires contact with the Executive Director/CEO or equivalent in the organization. One of the difficulties within complex multi-layered organizations is that decision-making often resides with a number of different professional groups and/or administrators. Ideally, the key senior personnel have already been informed and can link the researcher and/or research team with the relevant personnel.

When planning, developing and improving healthcare services, specific populations within the health service can provide valuable feedback about the delivery of the service. These clearly defined population groups, such as oncology patients undergoing radiotherapy or day only surgical patients, are an important (and often popular) target group for researchers. In addition, these types of projects can clearly 'add benefit' to core business and are more likely to be viewed favourably and supported by health agencies.

---

### ! Hot Tip: Privacy issues when targeting certain groups

If the study involves contacting patients (and hence obtaining their addresses) prior to admission or after discharge, you will need to carefully check the privacy legislation in your country to establish whether this is possible. The chairperson on the ethics committee can often help in this regard.

---

Particular local personnel may have specific requests how and about when the research subjects are to be accessed. There is a prevailing ethos that medical staff 'own' the patient. While this is debatable, they are certainly the chief gate keeper to this population. Concerns by doctors and other health professionals may focus around interrupting patient flow or arousing fear and apprehension unnecessarily in a population group. It is important that you are clear about what you are asking and what it is you hope to achieve. Similarly, nursing staff should be consulted as accessing patients requires

**Part 2**

identification of the best time in the flow of daily activities. Nurses can flag potentially difficult scenarios and limitations in your approach, for example, times when patients are fatigued and unlikely to be keen to participate or staff meetings/forums when staff will be unavailable. Administrative staff can also assist with facilitating patient contact as they have local information about such situations, as the timing of patient's meals and when visitors usually arrive.

If you are seeking approval to access the staff of the organization for research purposes then the senior management for that group of staff needs to approve. You also need to link with direct line managers to optimize physical access. This generally entails that you discuss and explain the research to everyone who is involved at the clinical level. It is unlikely that just one person in the health service will be able to provide you with all the requisite information to access your potential participants. So try and link up with as many associated personnel as possible.

## ! Hot Tip: Linking to your target population

Actively identify all personnel who may come in contact with your target population. Identify and establish the most suitable communication processes for each group of personnel. Remember: clinical staff usually do not prioritize answering their emails!

## ▶ Recruitment of research subjects

Now the strengths of your team building will be tested as you seek timely access to potential participants. If you do not have a local staff member on your team, you will need to call on your sponsor and champion to promote the project to the work area.

## ! Hot Tip: Offering staff incentives

Offering an incentive through a staff development opportunity and/or acknowledgement in the final publication can be powerful in motivating a local supporter. Be aware when seeking nurses' participation for staff surveys; most nurses are over the chocolate incentive!

You, as the researcher or as a member of the research team, can generally not be present for 24 hours of the day. The more that you inform staff and patients, and if they understand and support the aims of the research, there is greater likelihood that your recruitment process will be successful.

This preparatory work is essential in establishing recruitment processes whereby all potential participants can be approached. For example, in a study measuring the impact of discharge information for surgical patients, the surgical pre-admission lists and admissions through the emergency department were initially accessed. Daily visits to the surgical areas to access these patients identified another group of eligible patients that were on 'private' lists, that is, patients admitted 'privately' who were not anticipated admissions. These patients, not on a designated admission list, were identified through daily interactions with the Nurse Unit Managers (NUMs) in charge of the surgical units (Henderson and Zernike 2001). As the NUMs were supportive of the project, they were accepting of committing 5–10 minutes of their time each morning to identify eligible participants.

You will find that you have to explain the research and the information you require repeatedly to personnel in the local area during the data collection process! In a complex organization embedding any practice is difficult and unless the data collection phase continues over many months, it is unlikely to become embedded in day-to-day practice. Successful researchers become adept at explaining who they are and the when, what and how of their research quickly so that they can expediently enter the clinical area and access the information they need to locate potential research subjects without disrupting clinical staff and routines.

## ! Hot Tip: Communicating your research

Determine a couple of simple, clear statements that succinctly explain your research in a non-threatening way to clinical staff. Practise these with a precise request about your immediate needs: clinicians as busy people are often keen to expedite your requests.

### ▶ When timing is crucial

Access to timely information requires that you or a member of the research team constantly liaise with relevant personnel 'on the ground', for example, an admissions centre to identify prospective participants. In cases such as this, it is imperative that you link with the key personnel in

Part 2

the area that you are liaising. It is also helpful if the person(s)-in-charge of these areas are familiar with what type of information you require, for example, a patient's name and their reason for admission.

Of course, there are significant limitations about the information that can be given in these circumstances because of privacy laws. While personal information can not be disclosed, you and/or the research team can be notified that staff are commencing and a strategy provided to link with them, for example, when and where the scheduled orientation is to be conducted. Similarly, when staff resign they can be asked whether they agree for their name to be forwarded to an independent research team that interview staff at the cessation of their employment (Flint *et al.* 2006).

## Hot Tip: Establish a clear communication pathway

Experiment with developing the simplest but most reliable communication pathway between the area the participant group is located and the researcher to ensure the timeliness of information.

Timing is also a crucial factor when exploring specific patient interventions or stages of the illness trajectory. When this is the case, you need to clearly plan access to participants. If patients need to be accessed at 'crucial time periods', it is best to introduce the research to the prospective participants and gain consent for the periods that data will be collected at the outset. Organizing patient or staff consent and explaining the whole process to them at the commencement is not just necessary ethically (refer Chapter 2); it can facilitate timely access later when you meet with participants as they know what to expect. This can expedite data collection at a potentially busy time when you are collecting and collating data from a number of different areas.

Strong clinical links are needed if you are to be effective in accessing staff and patients at particular time periods. Studies where timing is critical, for example, the usefulness of discharge information for patients (Henderson and Zernike 2001), decision-making in terminal illness (Barry and Henderson 1996), and staff development interventions (Eaton *et al.* 2007), require an 'insider' (ideally a related staff member cognizant about clinical care delivery) as part of your research team. This team member will assist you with strategies for participant recruitment that need to be developed specific to the situation.

## ! Hot Tip: A team approach to data collection

Try and use the same team to make contact and collect data in the clinical area.

## ▶ Discharge information

When there is a need to access participants during a crucial time period, for example patients within the 24 hours prior to discharge (Henderson and Phillips 1996; Henderson and Zernike 2001), frequent regular visits to the designated ward areas is essential. The time of discharge, while supposedly planned in advance, is often only confirmed within the 24-hour period prior to departure. The more detailed knowledge the team has of patient flow and procedures, the more they can streamline research work and maximize capture of potential participants.

## ▶ Decision-making during the illness trajectory

Longitudinal studies (often undertaken in patient populations) benefit greatly from the commitment and constancy of clinical staff to alert you and the research team to readmissions and/or critical episodes. If this is not able to be attained, extensive resources can be expended on appropriate occasions to seek patients. A pilot study exploring cancer patients' decision-making preference during the illness trajectory was plentiful in the richness of the data collected: this was possible because of the Clinical Nurse Consultant (CNC) situated in the ward area. The CNC was aware of participating patients' specific situation; that is, scheduled outpatient appointments and readmissions. This knowledge of the patient enabled the researchers to identify pertinent times along the illness trajectory to undertake interviews (Barry and Henderson 1996).

## ! Hot Tip: Alerts for potential participants

Trial different triggers during the preparation stage to alert the data collectors to potential participants.

Part 2

## ▶ The value and limitations of databases

Eventually, staff and patient movements are recorded on databases. However, in many instances the research question requires that patients are approached as an inpatient just prior to discharge (Henderson and Zernike 2001) or staff are approached on their departure (Flint *et al.* 2006). While databases can provide an extensive data set, in clinical research where a particular episode of care or situation is being investigated the database maybe of limited value. In clinical care episodes, mechanisms and processes need to be in place that alert you and/or the research team to potential participants prior to being lodged on the database. Databases are useful in recording and storing large sets of information pertaining to specific patient or staff groups and/or specific incidents. In situations, as just explained, where the information is needed prior to the entry into the database, the database can be useful in cross checking total numbers.

The quality of any database is dependent on the veracity of the information that has been entered. When collecting information from participants, it is important that you seek the information directly from the participant. If information from a database is used then this should be cross checked with the participant. Clinical audits are often managed by large databases. In these situations, it is important that there is clarity in the definitions of the data that is being inputted into the database. As clinical audits are often used across organizations for benchmarking, it is absolutely essential that each organization is using the same criteria and definitions for categorizing the data as comparisons will be of little value.

### Check List: Useful databases

☑ Consensus about definitions of what is being measured and how it is measured
☑ A pertinent range of measures related to the incident/profile that information is collected to assist in enhancing understanding about the situation being assessed
☑ Reliability between the data collection officers
☑ Restricting access to designated coders

## ▶ Planning the amount of time in the field: deliberations and considerations

When planning the time in the field, you need to reflect on whether there is greater value in maximizing the numbers of the response, or alternatively, is there value in restricting numbers and focusing on the quality of the data that will be collected. Exploring the context is an opportunity to reflect on this again. (This would have previously been a major consideration when deciding on the method for your research study.) Remember, any significant changes to your protocol need to be approved by the Human Research Ethics Committee.

A major consideration for when you are planning the time period for recruitment is the size of the sample required for your study in relation to the potential population. The power of the study is calculated before the study commences. Adequate power means that there are enough subjects to detect a difference in the question that you are studying. It informs you of the number of participants required to ensure that statistical significance is attained. Further consideration needs to be given to the numbers of potential participants that need to be approached to obtain sufficient numbers that will complete the research activities.

When considering the size of the sample to approach, consideration needs to be given to

1. the number of participants who will fit the criteria,
2. the number of participants who will decline the offer to participate,
3. the number of participants who will be able to be followed through after giving their consent.

While the ideal sample is a random sample for quantitative research (and this is the assumption of parametric tests), often clinical research because of practical issues accesses a convenience sample (Aitken *et al.* 2003). The use of convenience samples and entire populations are popular in clinical settings because of difficulties and time in obtaining reasonable data sets. However, Williamson (2003) argues that the use of parametric tests in such circumstances misrepresents the results. Alternative techniques can overcome these limitations such as randomization and permutation tests (Williamson 2003).

Selecting the sample for participants of qualitative research does not appear as prescriptive as for quantitative research. However, careful planning is necessary for this group of participants to guarantee 'useful' material that is rich in its content. The literature will provide you with some clues

Part 2

about numbers (research texts and also studies that are similar to yours). Generally, if quite specific groups are targeted then insights can be gleaned from small numbers of interviews and/or focus groups. The data collection process needs to continue until dominant paradigms/themes emerge.

## ▶ Maximizing retention: trials and longitudinal studies

In the recruitment of participants for trials and longitudinal studies the interest is not just in maximizing the numbers of participants consenting but rather sustaining their interest for continued participation in the clinical trial or research project.

The following from Aitken *et al.* (2003) provides a comprehensive list of the details that should be obtained after the participants consent at the time of recruitment:

- Full name of participant (including maiden name, married name, aliases)
- Address
- Phone number plus convenient contact times
- Birth date and birth place
- Physical description: racial/ethnic background
- Educational, occupational history
- Employment contact details
- Rehabilitation plans on discharge from hospital (e.g., staying with sister)
- Vacation plans
- Contact details of 2–3 people who have regular contact with the participant.
- General practitioner or other healthcare personnel whom the patient regularly visits.

Such information can be invaluable when following up 'lost' participants and maximizing retention from the recruitment.

## ▶ Summary

This chapter has emphasized how to enhance recruitment and reduce time wasted in this activity. In maximizing the best use of time it is useful to be mindful of the perspective of the clinicians. Increasing goodwill (as we noted in Chapter 1) and sustaining interest can go a long way to enhancing identification, location, access and recruitment of participants. The following checklist provides an overview of how to achieve this:

---

### Check List: Securing a population for the research

☑ Identify the population that can answer the question.
☑ Locate where this population is situated.
☑ Undertake surveillance of the area to identify the ebb and flow of events and participants.
☑ Strategically link with the key personnel in the organization to reach this population.
☑ Establish clear communication pathways during the data collection phase to maximize recruitment and retention of participants.

---

In Chapter 1 we explained that positive attitudes of staff, patients and other significant people in the area towards the research is more likely when the researcher(s) visiting the area remain relatively constant. Too many different personnel associated with the research can create confusion for the staff in the area. When local staff are informed and involved, then they can be keen to assist. Nurse Unit Managers, who largely co-ordinate the healthcare team, are often pivotal in assisting with access as they are particularly knowledgeable about patient populations and profiles, together with healthcare routines and activities.

Similar to intervention studies where the 'site' for the intervention needs to be carefully planned and organized, consideration needs to be given to the logistics of where, how and when surveying, focus groups and interviews are progressed after the population has been recruited. It is these logistics that we focus upon in Chapter 6.

### ▶ References

Aitken, L., Gallagher, R. and Madronio, C. (2003). Principles of recruitment and retention in clinical trials. *International Journal of Nursing Practice*, 9: 338–46.

Barry, B. and Henderson, A. (1996). Nature of decision-making in the terminally ill patient. *Cancer Nursing*, 19(5): 384–91.

Part 2

Eaton, A., Henderson, A. and Winch, S. (2007). Enhancing nurses' capacity to facilitate learning in nursing students: effective dissemination and uptake of best practice guidelines. *International Journal of Nursing Practice*, 15(3): 316–20.

Flint, A., Webster, J., Fleming, L., Courtney, M. and Mason, T. (2006). Line managers perceptions of why staff leave – are they the same? Presented at Nursing Leadership in a Changing World: Bring it on. Association of Queensland Nurse Leaders (Inc) Conference, September, Brisbane, Australia.

Henderson, A. and Phillips, S. (1996). Surgical patients' information needs on discharge: are they being met? *International Journal of Nursing Practice*, 2(4): 229–35.

Henderson, A. and Zernike, W. (2001). A study of the impact of discharge information for surgical patients. *Journal of Advanced Nursing*, 35(3): 1–7.

Walker, R. (2006). The meaningful experiences of being an RN Buddy involved in undergraduate clinical nursing education. Unpublished Masters Thesis. School of Nursing and Midwifery, Griffith University, Brisbane.

Williamson, G.R. (2003). Misrepresenting random sampling? A systematic review of research papers in the Journal of Advanced Nursing. *Journal of Advanced Nursing*, 44(3): 278–88.

# Chapter six

# The hard work begins: maximizing participation

*Amanda Henderson and Linda Shields*

## Contents

The exponential growth of research within health care coupled with the demand for greater accountability has led to an explosion of research and evaluation in health care. Given this situation, some healthcare-based populations feel 'over researched' and have become disinterested in participating and contributing to research. In order for your project to succeed, it must be effectively marketed and the methods of data collection maximized to ensure the best response. Good response rates and quality responses are the backbone of a well designed and planned project, and obviously make a difference in the strength of your conclusions and subsequent publication.

Part 2

## ▶ Gaining traction – 'marketing the research'

A marketing strategy is vital to the success of your project. Research participants are increasingly discerning in health care. The expectation that most staff or patients will participate in your proposed research is an attitude of the past. Many individuals are aware of their rights, including their right not to participate. Increasingly, research teams need to consider the following: What can we offer participants? Why would individuals (staff, patients or carers) want to participate in this research?

Typically, research consent forms explain that while there may not be any direct benefit to the participant in the study, there is potentially a benefit to future populations. This almost altruistic notion that accompanied participation in research is no longer a sustainable draw card to attract participants. 'Marketing', that buzz word that is now unavoidable in everyday life, becomes paramount even to researchers! Ideally, 'marketing' provides a strategy for you, the researcher(s), to engage an otherwise disinterested potential participant group.

Marketing, of course, largely depends on the research, namely, the research question under investigation and the method being used. You and the team need to identify the 'hook' that will inspire the potential participant group. In Chapter 1 we spoke of framing the research in terms of organizational needs. Now we need to frame the research in terms of value for the participants.

---

## ! Hot Tip: Identifying the hook for participants

- ☑ Motivation
- ☑ Interest
- ☑ Personal and/or professional gain

---

## ▶ Marketing the research to the population

If you have invested time in the planning process, including discussing the project with the organization, maximizing participation is easier through co-operation of local personnel. We have noted that if the constituents of the clinical area get a good 'feel' for the research, they will support it through facilitating the research team access to potential participants. This will assist in promoting your research to prospective research subjects.

When considering the range of data collection methods (surveys, focus groups or interviews), the question needs to be balanced between the *value* of the response with the *likelihood* of response.

## ▶ Health facility staff as participants

Staff surveys are often viewed by clinicians as being inconsequential to their work. Clinicians tire of being 'subjects of study'; and surveys distributed to clinical staff are frequently dismissed without even being read. The challenge for any research project is for a reasonable response rate – while research texts will offer information about what constitutes a reasonable response rate (Parahoo 2006), not as much consideration is given to how this response rate is achieved.

Two factors directly impact on the numbers of responses. First, you need to maximize the distribution, and second, enhance return rate. Circulating surveys attached to pay sheets is a successful method to increase the distribution and consequently the number of surveys disseminated. Yet, as this method lacks the 'personal touch', response rates can be low because there is limited opportunity for potential participants to engage with you to establish the importance of the project and encourage their participation, for example, staff on extended leave will receive the survey but are most probably not interested in responding as their work may not be in their immediate interest. Distribution attached to pay sheets needs to be preceded by extensive communication, supported by a local champion, and targeted at staff 'active' in the workforce to improve the response rate.

Another strategy is targeting only the clinicians working during the current roster period. In a study exploring nurses' intention to treat a hypothetical patient's pain only 90% of the nurses on the roster were targeted, as these represented the nurses who were working a shift during the data collection period of the study. This was deemed appropriate to enhance response rate as the researcher involved in the data collection visited the nurses in the clinical area to remind them about the research and ask them to consider completing the survey that they had received in the internal mail. However, management needs to agree to this initiative as it may irritate some staff (Horbury *et al.* 2005).

Health practice, in particular nursing, is largely an oral culture and this can be a significant determinant in the attitudes that are formed about research conducted in the clinical area (Horder 2004). Discussing your project with potential participants in the local area is a strategic way to draw on the oral culture to develop interest in your research.

Part 2

---

### ! Hot Tip: Understanding the nature of your target group

Try to understand the nature of the behaviour of your target group so that you can effectively maximize the response from this group.

---

Staff meetings provide an obvious opportunity for information about the research to be verbally communicated and for staff to voice any concerns in a larger forum. If you intend to survey the staff, indicate how you are going to distribute the surveys or where the surveys will be left. This strategy will not leave staff feeling coerced or 'under pressure' to complete the survey as they can decide in their own time if they want to complete the survey.

Surveys are more popular when they are short. A 10-page survey used to measure nurses' intention to treat patients' pain was perceived by staff as long and repetitive, arguably the reason for only a 24.9% response rate despite the follow-up (Horbury *et al.* 2005). Unfortunately, this was necessary to assess the question under investigation.

Alternatively, a one-page format has proved popular where the demographic information is on the front and the questions fit into the centre page. While the limitation of this format is that the font can be small if there are many questions, and unsuitable for many in-patient groups, this is often not problematic for staff and students groups who are adept at reading small print. This format can be fairly quickly completed by staff and student groups.

---

### ! Hot Tip: Take care with the presentation of the survey

For staff groups try and make the survey form a little 'jazzy' – try and inject some interest in the format and presentation. Also make it 'snappy' – quick and to the point.

---

### Making surveys positive to staff

While surveys are over utilized and staff tire of them, they do have the ability to be quickly analysed. This can mean fairly rapid feedback to the participants. A 'quick' turn around is ideal as surveys are not left taking up space in clinical areas and do not become a 'bore' or a 'nuisance'. Also, it is more likely that feedback to participants is timely and therefore meaningful as many of the staff can recall the survey and the circumstances that existed at the time of its distribution. Clinical staff can have high turnover rates. Giving prompt feedback means there is a greater chance that the findings are indicative of the particular population that is receiving the results. If the turn around period is protracted, in situations such as workforce culture surveys, the personnel dynamics in the area may have changed. Consequently, staff may have no knowledge of the survey when the findings are presented, and therefore the survey will hold little meaning for them.

---

! **Hot Tip: Identifying the significance of the survey content to staff**

Include statements such as . . . 'we (the research team) have had discussions about the significance of this issue with management. The intention of the research is to provide clarity on . . . (mention a specific issue) so that effective mechanisms can be recommended'.

---

Information to staff participants that indicates relevant members of the organization are interested in the research findings to inform changes carries a powerful message to staff.

If the management team of the organization does feedback to participants about survey results and discusses changes that have been adopted because of the findings, this can act as a catalyst for greater involvement 'next time around' where staff maybe encouraged to be involved because of positive outcomes.

### Staff participation in interviews and focus groups

Focus groups and interviews are potentially very informative. They are often used in the exploratory stages of research to identify a range of issues that relate to a problem and also can provide a description of the issues.

Attendances by staff at focus groups and also interviews can be notoriously low. A longitudinal study seeking feedback from new graduates at a large tertiary teaching hospital had only 16 new graduate participants in focus groups when invited at 2–3 months after employment. This reduced

**Part 2**

to 12 participants when focus groups were conducted 6–9 months after the new graduates commencement date (Fox *et al*. 2005). This was from a potential population of over 100 new graduates who commenced their employment at the organization.

---

! **Hot Tip: Seek an interesting angle to the focus group**

As many topics hold little interest to clinicians, ascertain whether focus groups will attract a good response – if at all possible try and make an interesting slant to the focus group – possibly pose a question in the advertisement.

---

Focus groups and interviews are more successful when they pertain to interest areas for staff, for example, 'hot topics' where staff desire to share their thoughts and ideas. There is always a problem if the focus group or interview is on a topic that holds little interest to the clinician. In a recent study (Walker 2006), very few clinicians nominated to be interviewed about their experiences of working with undergraduate students, as generally working with students does not generate much interest with clinicians.

Selling the purpose of the focus group or interview, what it is going to achieve and the benefits to the individual(s) can motivate individuals to participate. Ideally for focus groups and interviews, the leadership and management team should provide time for staff to be released. The researcher(s) need to negotiate with the management team the cost of backfill for staff and include this in their budget.

---

! **Hot Tip: 'Backfilling' staff to increase participation**

For maximum participation negotiate payment for 'backfill' time for staff and commence advance planning for rostering. Securing funds so that clinical staff can participate in the research in work time can still be difficult if there is insufficient qualified staff to relieve. In our experience, participation rates will be poor if you conduct interviews and focus groups in the participant's time.

---

## Increasing participation in focus groups

Focus groups can be an invaluable forum for staff to raise issues of greatest concern to them, especially, if participants derive some sense of collegiality when they recognize that they are not alone in their concerns. The chance to share thoughts means that focus groups can potentially be sold as a 'feel good' opportunity. If access can be arranged through normal meeting times then gaining participation in focus groups is generally not difficult if the topic is of interest to staff.

A successful strategy for increasing participation has been the timing and location of focus groups. In a study seeking feedback about the value of establishing a Clinical Development Unit, focus groups were carefully timed to coincide with regular meetings and located within the ward area. Focus groups were conducted during the period in the early afternoon when the scheduled morning and afternoon shifts 'overlapped'. This time was selected to maximize attendance. All nurses working on both shifts were invited to attend the focus groups. This resulted in a total of 29 registered nurses providing feedback which represented 43% of the staff who worked in the area (Henderson *et al.* 2007).

## Hot Tip: Timing is everything!

Identify the best time in the clinician's busy day to get access. We have found that 11 a.m. is often most suitable or change over of shifts, if there is an extended period where the shifts overlap.

When focus groups bring together individuals who may not know each other starting discussion maybe slow. Ideally, participants are provided with food and drink and an atmosphere that is conducive to wanting to stay and take part. The value of an experienced facilitator is paramount in these situations. The facilitator of the focus group needs a dynamic demeanour as sometimes it can be difficult to 'get the group going'.

It can be difficult to draw individuals into the focus group at the requisite time. Cascading continuous information such as notices, phone calls or one-on-one visits remind participants and assist them to know that their contribution is important and highly sought. If you are unable to gain enough participants for your focus group then it can be useful to undertake an interview format. In a longitudinal study exploring preceptor's perceptions of an education program and organizational support, four focus

Part 2

groups were conducted at the second time period with six, one-on-one interviews to maximize participation (Henderson *et al.* 2006). Combining focus group and interview methods facilitated a reflective process that arose from the same set of questions. This was congruent with the researcher's aim of eliciting experiential insights that would provide a greater depth of information than that obtained from surveys (Henderson *et al.* 2006).

### Making the interview successful

Interviews are usually time-consuming. The following checklist can help you get the most out of your interview.

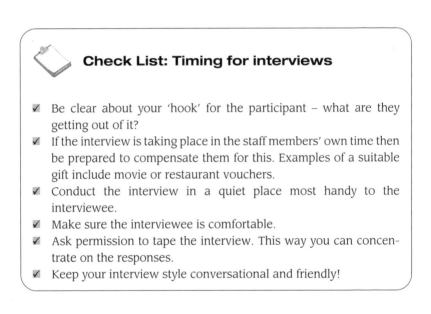

### Check List: Timing for interviews

☑ Be clear about your 'hook' for the participant – what are they getting out of it?

☑ If the interview is taking place in the staff members' own time then be prepared to compensate them for this. Examples of a suitable gift include movie or restaurant vouchers.

☑ Conduct the interview in a quiet place most handy to the interviewee.

☑ Make sure the interviewee is comfortable.

☑ Ask permission to tape the interview. This way you can concentrate on the responses.

☑ Keep your interview style conversational and friendly!

### An over-researched population: the example of nurses

The largest percentage of the health professional workforce and a significant influence on work practices and culture within the health industry, nurses are targeted as subjects of research studies by many health professional groups such as psychologists, allied health professionals and administrators. Nurses are now in danger of becoming an over researched group (Pittman 1989). While research that focuses on clinical issues relevant to nursing are now an acceptable and growing area of research, the obsession with surveying, interviewing and conducting focus groups continues unabated with the nursing workforce.

## ! Hot Tip: Survey only those you need

Prior to embarking on large-scale staff surveys, critically examine your rationale. Studying particular cohorts (units with high turnover or reduced absenteeism), which can be identified through Human Resource Management databases, maybe more useful to your purposes.

## ▶ Patients and carers as participants

### Patient participation in surveys, focus groups and interviews

Patients and their carers can be a very different proposition to staff in health facilities in their desire to give of their time to participate in the research that is being undertaken. Traditionally, patients have readily given of their time to complete surveys or undertake interviews. However, uninterrupted time in a hospital bed is diminishing with shorter lengths of stay in hospitals, increasing patient acuity and more interventions and procedures.

Naturally, a patient's willingness to accept or decline to participate in research is affected by their well-being. Difficulties with patient recruitment may be experienced in a variety of populations. A study into patient's information needs on admission to a rehabilitation study resulted in only 9 out of 15 patients being eligible during the study period. This is because the exclusion criteria, namely, diagnosis of dementia, a psychiatric co-morbidity, a current acute illness, aphasia and a mini-mental score of below 24, ruled out many participants (McKain *et al.* 2005). Furthermore, if patients are experiencing pain and lethargy as part of recovering from major surgery or trauma, or alternatively malaise from medical conditions, they are unlikely to be motivated to consent to participate in research studies.

## ! Hot Tip: Think about your inclusion and exclusion criteria

Take care with your inclusion and exclusion criteria for participant recruitment. Are these critical to answering your research question? If strict criteria is necessary then make sure your recruitment period is long.

Part 2

The experience of accessing information from patients is different from health facility staff. For example, surveys that are often quick for staff to interpret and respond to may take much longer for patient or carer populations. Often the reason for this is simple factors, such as patients needing their 'reading' glasses, and these not being available, or not able to be worn, because of tubes or dressings. In many cases admission to hospital is already associated with significant amounts of 'literature' regarding what to expect, the routine, and arrangements prior to discharge. In these cases the completion of yet another form (your survey) may not hold much interest for them.

When approaching patients with a survey form, you can use other 'getting to know you' strategies that may assist in developing a rapport with them. Clinicians who undertake studies drawing on patients within their specialized field can often talk broadly to the patient about what is known about the patient's condition and share this general knowledge with the patient.

NOTE: While this is a good opportunity to establish rapport, discussions need to be undertaken with the clinical staff in the unit about 'boundaries' or 'caveats' around the information given.

## ! Hot Tip: Establish a rapport with your patient

Rather than just approach patients with a questionnaire – try to gain some sense of their needs, for example, are they tired, bored, in need of something or prefer to be left alone? If the situation permits, an offer of a drink can be received positively by the patient.

### Overcoming recruitment barriers with patients

To overcome some of the difficulties with surveys, you can chose a more interactive method of data collection such as interviews or focus groups with patients.

### Patients and interviews

Patients of a reasonable health status who may find completing a survey challenging (or boring!) may be happy to participate in an interview. Depending on the stage of their illness, many patients can appreciate the opportunity to talk about their illness and their care. If you have developed a questionnaire, this can form the structure of your interview. Be prepared to listen to issues that are peripheral to the research as well as the responses to the relevant questions – this assists in building rapport. A positive experience by one patient that is communicated to others can facilitate the recruitment of others.

## ⚠ Hot Tip: Allow plenty of time for interviewing

Patients often enjoy talking about the history around their hospitalization – be prepared to gather large amounts of information that may seem peripheral to your research. As patients are not always fully cognizant of your particular intent, it may take a little time to explain the aim and rationale of your particular study.

An open-ended interview (ideally taped) with sufficient time allowed can be an invaluable source of rich information that may inform later studies. For example, a study exploring cancer patient's desire for participation in decision-making, identified the degree to which patients wanted to participate in decision-making on the initial palliative care admission and along the illness trajectory. What also emerged was another set of data that suggested that patients desired greater participation as they 'learnt more' about their illness (Barry and Henderson 1996).

Of course, eliciting such information from patients can be very time-consuming. When accessing information from patients through questionnaires or interviews, it is important that the researcher does not have other commitments within a short time frame for two reasons. First, because patients can possibly have many questions about the research (therefore consenting is time-consuming) and, second, many peripheral issues maybe raised when the patients respond to the question(s) posed to them.

### Focus groups for 'outpatients' or 'interest groups'
Focus groups are usually not an option for patients in acute tertiary facilities because many are not mobile or available at the same time. Where focus groups can be useful is with patient groups who meet outside of the hospital ward such as an outpatients' clinic or a support group. Access to these patient populations provides a wealth of information. The difficulty is accessing these participants in an ethical manner. Such groups can be hesitant of 'outsiders' visiting – for example, researchers who are

**Part 2**

often perceived as 'grabbing and running': they direct questions to obtain information pertinent to their needs but do not contribute to the emotional well being of the group.

Patients can be reticent about research and its opportunities. A number of participants with multiple sclerosis in the first stage of a survey did not elect to take up free consultation and advice from an incontinence adviser as part of the second stage of the project, even though they reported experiencing incontinence issues. While a number of these people reported that they were 'okay', the researchers concluded that if the community was aware of the assistance an incontinence adviser could offer then they would more likely take up this opportunity (Wollin *et al.* 2005).

---

## ! Hot Tip: Finding the hook for participation

Prior to communicating with these groups, identify your 'hook'. Try to ensure that it is the hook you are able to deliver on! Make sure you give something back to the group, be that your findings, a poster or an education session!

---

## ▶ Accessing carers

One group of potential participants who may be of value in your study are 'carers'. These individuals spend considerable amounts of time waiting alongside the patient as they undergo procedures or sleep. They often have more free time than the patient and are able to observe routines and practices. In hospital terms, carers are attached to patients and permission to approach the carer is usually gained from the patient's medical officer to approach the patient and then the carer. If you are not sure how to recruit carers then approach the chairperson of the ethics committee.

## ▶ Use of secondary records and archive information

During data collection, often data other than that designed to be included in the analysis are collected. Sometimes, it may be possible to use this data for further analysis, or the data itself might suggest some other way of beginning a completely new research project. If the project is different from the original study, ethical approval needs to be sought for the new part of the study.

Secondary data can provide great opportunities for extra investigation; for example, in a study of the needs of parents of hospitalized children, information about the costs to the parents of parking at the hospital and the cost of hospital meals was collected. This enabled a second study which highlighted how difficult hospital stays could be for parents on low incomes (Shields and Tanner 2004). A drug trial will yield data about the drug on trial, but may also demonstrate previously unknown reactions in the human body. Never be scared to use secondary data, but remember, if the new study is similar to the original study for which ethical approval was given, then the secondary study can go ahead. If it is entirely different, then further ethical approval will be needed.

### Making the most of searching archives

Data stored in archives provides a useful source of information for researchers. This type of research is something of an art form, as it can be complex, frustrating, tedious, always time-consuming, and requires a different set of skills to those needed for clinical research. However, it can be very rewarding and extremely interesting to do.

### ! Hot Tip: Staying focused in archival studies

Stay focused! Archival studies contain a trap for the researcher: in browsing through archives, no matter how determined one may be to stay focused on the specific data one wants to collect, it is ever so easy to become completely engrossed in all the available data.

An epidemiological project that examined patterns of growth in children at an Aboriginal community in Australia used baby health clinic records to collect birth weights at different ages of children over three generations of several families (Alsop-Shields 1997). There was other fascinating information about feeding methods and advice given to mothers by the infant welfare nurse 30–40 years ago. Of course, these topics warranted further research projects. Diligence was mandatory to stay focused on collecting the data about the babies' weights.

Part 2

Archival records are often used for history projects, but can be used for a variety of investigations, for example, department and criminal court records to investigate levels of child abuse in a particular population, or department of education records to explore the effects of teenage pregnancy on school performance. These are but a few examples, but for all such projects, there are a few basic rules.

1. Before you start, examine the archive thoroughly to make sure it contains what you want, and that the records are complete, or at least have few gaps.
2. Make sure you obtain the correct permission. If you are unsure about how to do this and what is required, ask the person responsible for the archive, who may be an archivist, a librarian or maybe the chairperson of the committee to whom the archive belongs.
3. Before you begin data collection, familiarize yourself with the archive, its forms and what they contain. Develop a data collection sheet, and trial it before you begin; in other words, have a 'dummy run' and collect the data you need from a small number of records from the archive. If there are problems with your data collection sheet, you can fix it.
4. Make sure your research question is sound, and can be answered using the data in the archive. It is both inefficient and frustrating if you get halfway through your study and find that what you are looking at is not what you set out to investigate.
5. When you write the paper or thesis from your archival project, always thank (in the 'acknowledgments' section) the owners of the archive, the librarian or archivist who helped you find the data or gave you access to the records, and anyone else who was involved in helping you get the most out of the archival records.

▶ **Observation: less demanding on participants?**

Observation is not demanding of any particular participant's time: apart from the consent required from the participant to be observed, there maybe no other requirement. However, while it may not be time-consuming for participants, it can be very time-consuming for the researcher because of the logistics of observation. To identify significant situations/record prevalence of particular activities or describe situations for the generation of common meanings and/or phenomena, considerable data needs to be collected.

Ethically, observation studies are fraught with difficulty. Traditionally, with observation studies as long as the organization approved the study it could continue. These assumptions have now changed with each individual requiring to consent before being able to be observed – the logistics of this can be difficult in a busy dynamic healthcare setting where many participants enter and leave on a once only basis (and often very briefly at that). A strategy used more recently in an observation study was that only those practices pertaining to participants who consented were used in the analysis and documentation of the research (Henderson *et al.* in press).

---

### ! Hot Tip: Determine your strategy for participant consent during observation at the outset

As observation work can potentially be fraught with ethically challenging situations – identify a clear path of how ethical consent is going to be obtained from the participant population. Furthermore, a clear decision tree needs to be developed about dealing with particular ethical issues as they arise. This should be negotiated with the Chair of the Ethics committee.

---

Careful negotiations and discussion are required with the clinical team to establish where and how to situate the observer as researcher. Good communication is needed to explain the general intent of the research so that staff do not become alarmed about the presence of a researcher.

Nurses are recognized as being suitable researchers within the clinical context to undertake observation studies. Arguably, there is an ease of 'fitting in' because of nurses' familiarity with the environment (Savage 1995). However, it is imperative that the theoretical position of the nurse is clearly established prior to the observation period because the position adopted by the nurse researcher affects every phase of the study from the way the question is constructed to the final presentation of the results (Borbasi *et al.* 2005). Once this has been articulated, it will guide how and where the researcher is situated, the use of data collection strategies such as videoing, taping or field notes, the amount of exposure and time in the area, all of which needs to be communicated and organized with the local team.

Part 2

## ▶ Intervention studies: a competitive edge

In our experience staff often do not get feedback that is useful to them regarding research. Even when feedback is forthcoming then there is still little guarantee that anyone is going to act on the information. Intervention studies offer a tangible gain for the staff in the organization in relation to a perceived benefit in the form of instruction, training or support. Intervention studies can be well received by populations – they can also act as a source of staff development. While these perceived benefits can enhance motivation and participation, there are a number of limitations. Limitations for intervention studies in hospital-based clinical staff populations include:

1. Matching large numbers of part-time shift workers pre- and post-intervention;
2. The larger the size of the population for the intervention, the better possibility of demonstrating any differences; however, expanding the intervention creates difficulties regarding consistency in the approach and local work-based practices;
3. The constancy of clinical practice means that invariably all staff are unable to attend as in many areas clinical work cannot just be stopped;
4. Difficulty in identifying a tool that is sensitive enough to measure specific changes with an intervention.

A further limitation is that if these studies are rigorous in their approach, there is often a control group; and unfortunately one area needs to be in the control group and therefore not receive any intervention. Disappointment of staff groups that act as a control can be curtailed by discussion of crossover designs – this provides an opportunity for the intervention albeit in a delayed time frame. Intervention strategies are powerful in the enthusiasm that they develop for research. Good rapport can be developed.

## ▶ Making a difference through clinical research

Marketing usually involves incentives – we see them everyday – free coffee samples in the mail, the chance to win a digital camera or beachside holiday. Chocolates attached to survey forms and luring afternoon teas at focus groups are a reasonable start but increasingly these are of little interest to participants.

Gaining popularity are incentives in the form of immediate feedback. Online computer surveys can give you an immediate response on completion of the questionnaire in relation to your answer when compared with the surveys already received. In the clinical context this immediate response is difficult. However, the staff have to believe that feedback will inform future directions, and convincing staff about this can be very difficult when staff have become increasingly cynical and disenfranchised. Evidence of previous successes (if there are any) could be one way to tackle the cynicism.

## ▶ Summary

There are many data collection methods available for potential researchers, namely surveys, questionnaires, focus groups, interviews. In this chapter we have identified the best ways to use these in health facility clinical and staff populations. These considerations need to be examined quite closely with both the question and the proposed population to determine with confidence the best way to collect your data for maximum participation and quality that directly affects the worthiness of the findings.

## ▶ References

Alsop-Shields, L. (1997). The growth of children for two generations at an Australian Aboriginal Community. *Journal of Pediatric Nursing*, 11(6): 402–8.

Barry, B. and Henderson, A. (1996). Nature of decision-making in the terminally ill patient. *Cancer Nursing*, 19(5): 384–91.

Borbasi, S., Jackson, J. and Wilkes, L. (2005). Fieldwork in nursing research: positionality, practicalities and predicaments. *Journal of Advanced Nursing*, 51(5): 493–501.

Fox, R., Henderson, A. and Malko-Nyhan, K. (2005). 'They survive despite the organisational culture not because of it': A longitudinal study of new staff perceptions of what constitutes support during transition to an acute tertiary facility. *International Journal of Nursing Practice*, 11: 193–9.

Henderson, A., Fox, R. and Malko-Nyhan, K. (2006). An evaluation of preceptor's perceptions of educational preparation and organizational support for their role. *The Journal of Continuing Education in Nursing*, 37(3): 130–6.

Henderson, A., Boyde, M. and Winch, S. (2007). Assessing the impact of a clinical development unit in cardiology. *Contemporary Nurse*, 24(1): 25–32.

Henderson, A., van Eps, M., Pearson, K., James, C., Henderson, P. and Osborne, Y. (in press). 'Caring for' behaviours that indicate to patients

**Part 2**

that nurses 'care about' them. *Journal of Advanced Nursing*, manuscript number 2006-0638.

Horbury, C., Henderson, A. and Bromley, B. (2005). Influences of patient behaviour on clinical nurses' pain assessment: implications for continuing education. *The Journal of Continuing Education in Nursing*, 36(1): 18–24.

Horder, W. (2004). Reading and not reading in professional practice. *Qualitative Social Work*, 3(3): 297–311.

McKain, S., Henderson, A., Kuys, S., Drake, S., Kerridge, L. and Ahern, K. (2005). Exploration of patients' need for information on arrival at a geriatric and rehabilitation unit. *Journal of Clinical Nursing*, 14: 704–10.

Parahoo, K. (2006). *Nursing Research: Principles, Process and Issues*. Palgrave Macmillan, Basingstoke, UK.

Pittman, E. (1989). Making the most of new opportunities: clinical nursing research in the 1990s. In Gray, G. and Pratt, R. (eds) *Issues in Australian Nursing 2*, Churchill Livingstone, Melbourne.

Savage, J. (1995). *Nursing Intimacy: An Ethnographic Approach to Nurse-Patient Interaction*. Scutari Press, London.

Shields, L. and Tanner, A. (2004). Costs of meals and parking for parents of hospitalised children in Australia. *Paediatric Nursing*, 16(6): 14–18.

Walker, R. (2006). Masters dissertation. Griffith University, Australia.

Wollin, J., Bennie, M., Leech, C., Windsor, C. and Spencer, N. (2005). Multiple sclerosis and continence issues: an exploratory study. *British Journal of Nursing*, 14(8): 439–48.

# Part three
# Collecting data and disseminating findings

# Chapter seven

# Operationalizing the data collection

*Amanda Henderson and Kerri Holzhauser*

## ▶ Contents

All your 'leg work' should be completed at this stage. Now you can start collecting data from your newly recruited research participants. After all the preparatory work needed to gain support for your research, obtain ethics approval, secure funding and locate your subjects, this process possibly seems straightforward. However, you need a further set of strengths to effectively manage the collection of data. In many ways it can be likened to inventors who after they invent a piece of equipment set out in a different direction to manufacture and commercialize their invention. Now the research team directs its efforts to the logistics of systematically

Part 3

deriving the data from its source, sending it to your research office and organizing it in an accessible readily usable form to be used later for data analysis.

In your master proposal you will have devised a timeline that proposes time periods for specific tasks within the research process. It is not unusual for these timelines to 'blow out'. A constant theme throughout this book is always allow more time than initially anticipated. Some guidelines suggest that you at least triple or quadruple the anticipated time periods for tasks to be completed. The extension of timelines depends on many factors including, how long it takes to obtain funding and ethics approval, how realistic projections are for the recruitment of subjects, and the degree to which unforeseen workloads impinge on the time that the research team can commit to providing direction about processes and giving feedback about preliminary reports.

The following checklist will help you effectively operationalize your project.

---

### Check List: Getting the research moving!

☑ A planning document to co-ordinate the research process and remind you about the timing and type of communications.

☑ A log or a journal to record specific conversations and decisions, and so on as the project proceeds. This is particularly important if you make changes and have continuing communications between the funding and ethical bodies.

☑ A diary of issues that arise during data collection.

☑ A strategy for collecting and organizing the data regardless of whether it is in the form of surveys, focus groups, interviews or observations.

---

### ▶ Planning calendars (and task-tracking documents)

The planning document communicates to the whole team the progress of the research, from when the idea is conceptualized to the dissemination of results.

Establishing a clear (and ideally very noticeable) 'Planning Calendar' has the advantage of

- Making explicit to the team when, how and who is responsible for particular events integral to the research the planning of;
- Clear timelines for the recruitment and employment of staff to and within the research team (or reminder dates for yourself if you are attending to this);
- Visual reminder and an easy 'reckoner' of pertinent dates, for example when surveys need to be distributed, collected or when focus groups/interviews are being conducted;
- Keeping you updated of where the research is up to;
- Identifying when progress reports are due (often required by funding bodies);
- A record to return to when reporting on the research.

The use of something as simple as a calendar in the form of a large year planner can be useful. Distinctive symbols to highlight specific dates and background colours to indicate the stages of the research can give an easy to follow overall picture of the research. The Gantt chart you developed in your master proposal may now be refined. Specific dates that need to be obviously marked as important will be closing dates for funding submission, dates of key stakeholder group meetings or dates for feedback as requested by particular interested bodies. The following inclusions in a planning document can assist in co-ordinating team work and establishing timelines for the work of research assistants and/or data collectors, and considered times for the whole team (with or without stakeholders) to meet.

---

### Check List: Dates for your 'planning and tracking' document

- ☑ Final date for feedback on the research proposal
- ☑ Submission to ethics committee(s)
- ☑ Submission to sources of funding (closing dates for each source of funding)
- ☑ Advertisements to recruit staff
- ☑ Training of data collectors

**Part 3**

**Check List (Continued)**

☑ Dates of ongoing communication with clinical staff and other members of the research team to establish/confirm exact start date of data collection (and where necessary modifications to the proposal)

☑ Agreed dates and modes of communication between team members during data collection for updates

☑ Preparation and, where necessary, procurement of research materials, for example surveys, software/audio visual equipment (this needs to include appropriate education in the use of equipment)

☑ Dates for review of data collection processes to ascertain whether research is progressing as planned (before too much time and money is expended if significant modifications are needed)

Once the dates have been agreed and confirmed, then clarification (through email or a communication board) is needed about specific elements of the data collection process. When planning for data collection, the team needs to be clear about who is responsible for what research activities.

**Check List: For the allocation of research activities**

☑ Recruitment and consenting of research subjects
☑ Where relevant, follow-up of research subjects
☑ Distribution of surveys
☑ Collection of surveys
☑ Booking suitable rooms and facilities for interviews/focus groups
☑ Advertising and recruiting of participants for interviews/focus groups
☑ Focus group facilitation, taping and note taking
☑ Conducting of interviews
☑ The delivery of completed materials (whether surveys, focus group data, interviews) to the research team in accordance with ethical standards

At each stage of the research project the best form of communication (emails, letters or memos) should be sent to all members of staff providing an update. This communication should include a statement about the following:

- What stage of the research process is about to commence, for example advertising of staff, commencement of focus groups and the timeline for this 'subset' of the overall process;
- Who are the people involved at this stage;
- What the expectation is of these people, for example attendance at a meeting, preparation of an information poster or obtaining information;
- A request for a response (by when and the format) should be included.

## ! Hot Tip: Start recruiting staff early

Attend to the employment of staff early to ensure that you secure the staff best able to undertake the role you require. Advertising, short-listing, and organizing the date of commencement for research staff all need to be undertaken well in advance of the date required to participate in the research to ensure that the staff that you want (the staff most capable of undertaking the research work) are available. Because research work is generally not permanent work, qualified, capable staff, who can undertake the work that is required as part of the research, are usually already involved in other projects and/or clinical and academic work. Therefore time needs to be negotiated from the existing project or clinical or academic environments. With the increasing demand for expert clinicians, clinical areas are not in a position to release staff at short notice. Consequently, long lead in times are needed as the person you want is often an invaluable staff member where they are regularly employed.

## ▶ Employment of staff

Most projects will require employment of staff for certain tasks. You will have identified the number and type of staff in your master proposal and budget justification. Decisions about where these staff will be sourced need to be made, for example from the clinical area or from an academic area. You will also need to decide the mode of employment; that

Part 3

is, whether they will be part-time or casual employees, undertake second-ments or short-term contracts, and the awards will they be employed under.

You will need to collaborate with the manager(s) from the area(s) that staff are being released before the appointment and commencement details can be finalized. Once this has been secured, then emails, memos or letters (as well as the accompanying paperwork) can be forwarded to all the relevant personnel. Clear timeframes also need to be provided to the clinical area about when staff are likely to return. Where pos-sible, you should negotiate some flexibility around the accessibility of staff once they have returned to their clinical area, after their involvement with the research, as they can sometimes answer queries during the final report writing stage because of the domain of the research that they were involved.

## ▶ The use of a journal

A journal can be helpful in keeping a record of the progress, namely, the discussions and arrangements that you have made and therefore a record of how the logistics of the research may have altered slightly from what was initially planned; for example, a meeting with the out-patient department may mean that patients are approached before their visit to the doctor to ascertain their eligibility for recruitment as time available before the session is often much greater than the time afterwards.

Within the journal style log keep all copies of emails, letters and other correspondence between co-investigators, research assistants and other associated individuals. Keep notes of the jobs you have asked research assistants and support staff to do so you can easily keep a track of who does what, and if and when jobs are completed. Such rigorous attention to keeping notes will pay off during the write-up stage. Comprehensive notes mean there is little trouble in picking up where the project was left if there is a delay, or it may assist when reviewing why there are partial anomalies in the collection and analysis of data.

A journal is particularly useful in keeping notes about the discussions that occur around analysis of qualitative data. In the first instance everyone who undertakes analysis of narrative/descriptive data should analyse it independently. Everyone's accounts should be recorded and their rationale discussed. In the course of the journal the decisions collectively made by the group (including the rationale) should be documented so there is a clear understanding of the pathway that is progressed (more about analysis of data in Chapter 8).

## ▶ Collecting data: considerations in intervention studies

Keeping a journal is particularly important in intervention studies where the researcher should keep a record of the points mentioned in the following checklist.

---

### Check List: Intervention studies journal

☑  When the interventions took place
☑  The duration of the intervention
☑  The number of participants who attended or were exposed to the intervention (this should ideally include how many potential participants could have attended and reasons for their non-attendance)
☑  Any deviation to the intervention and why
☑  General comments from the participants combined with a summary by the facilitator of the session to record their impressions is useful when reflecting on the results

---

In an intervention study to examine the use of massage with music and aromatherapy in the management of stress and anxiety, nursing staff in the emergency department were randomly selected on two days of the week to undertake the intervention. During one of the two days when the massage intervention was planned, a helicopter crash occurred. As the primary importance for the emergency department was to effectively manage the multiple casualties as they arrived in the department, the research protocol was appropriately abandoned for that day. The research team recorded this deviation and documented comments in their data collection journal. The researchers referred to this deviation during the data analysis and dissemination stages of their project (Davis *et al.* 2005).

---

## ! Hot Tip: Deviating from protocols

If a deviation in protocol occurs, consider if the deviation needs to be reported to the Human Research Ethics Committee for consideration. Also refer to the Ethical Conduct of Human Research Guidelines in your country to determine when this should occur.

---

## ▶ Collecting data: considerations for focus groups

Facilitating focus groups can be a daunting task if you have little experience using qualitative methods of data collection. Before you start, have a clear outline of the questions you wish to ask and the information you aim to collect. Try to use open-ended questions that encourage participants to provide a detailed response. Asking yes/no questions does not encourage members of the group to provide their own ideas on a topic.

Core considerations for focus groups:

- Keep momentum;
- Promote fair participation;
- Stay on track;
- Probe beyond what is already known about the topic area under investigation;
- When an opinion is voiced, identify the prevalence of the opinion. For example, a participant in a study about new graduates transition to the workplace stated that they needed 'support'. While other participants agreed – the focus group leader determined the meaning of this comment and whether there was consistency about this meaning across the whole group (Fox *et al.* 2006).

In an attempt to gain equal participation by all members, observe participant's body language and attempts to contribute. If one person is monopolizing the conversation, direct your comment towards those ready to participate by using a bridging statement such as ' Mary, it appears you had something you wanted to add . . . '

Sometimes the discussions will bring up a variety of issues. Where possible, try to keep the conversations on a single topic of discussion. If another point of discussion arises during the conversation, make a brief note of the issue and when the issue being discussed has been covered, return to the previous point. A prompt you could use may be 'John, you mentioned facilitating learning before, could you please clarify what you meant'.

## Adding value to focus group findings

When you are conducting a focus group, it is virtually impossible to take notes and keep the conversations moving. Employing an experienced facilitator is beneficial to maximizing your results as you are free to observe and make an assessment of the non-verbal aspects of the process. All sessions should be taped for verification of data. If you need to write, keep the points very brief to remind you of issues you identify. At the first opportunity you have, preferably immediately after the focus group, write down a more detailed account of issues you feel are pertinent. You can check your notes against the tape later.

---

### ! Hot Tip: Recording responses from focus groups

In your master proposal you will have specified that you will record focus groups or interviews. Always ask participants prior to focus groups whether they consent to having the focus group taped. During the focus group try to refer to the participants by their name. It makes it easier when transcribing the recordings to identify prevalence of ideas by clarifying whose ideas belong to whom. When transcribing the focus groups, use a de-identified name such as Miss X or participant 1.

---

If you have a facilitator conducting the focus group for you, it can be useful to get feedback from the facilitator about their perceptions of the issues that may have been raised. This way you can avoid getting to the data analysis stage of the focus groups and discovering that perceptions have been identified but not explored.

### ▶ Collecting data in the field: recording observations on paper

It is a difficult task to accurately record 'field notes'. The more detail and explanation you can provide about when, where, how and what happened will give you greater clarity and assist with the authenticity in the interpretation. So often with field notes they are only legible to the recorder. In this case you need to re-write these within the first 24 hours to capture the depth and complexity of meaning, otherwise much of it may be forgotten. The re-writing of material is labour-intensive and consequently expensive.

In this section we suggest how to best organize the data recording sheets so that you and the research team can revisit the notes at a later time and make sense of all the material as it is recorded.

You need to organize field notes coherently from the outset. Record each session, how long and where in a book, inserting tabs from the start of each section (i.e., field experience).

The first page details the participants and your position (brief profile – but more importantly a coding system which can then be used to record further information).

Subsequent pages need to be organized to deal with the myriad and complexity of activities. In Figure 7.1 we demonstrate how to record observation data taken in a hospital ward. In Table 7.1 we show you how to

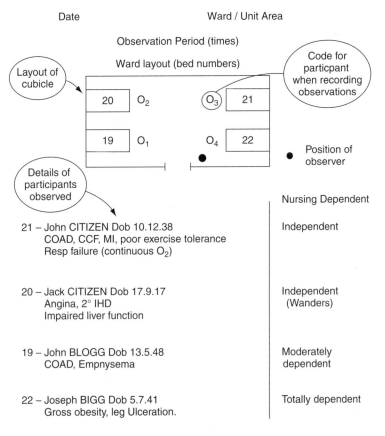

**Figure 7.1** *Recording data: ward layout and participants.*

**Table 7.1**  *Recording data: the participants and your observations*

| Time | Observed interactions | Observed behaviours | Comments and impressions (by the researcher) |
|---|---|---|---|
| 08:00 | To $O_3$ – Have you had a shower love? | Body language is respectful – tone is soft. | |
| | | Nurse makes the bed. | The nurse would appear not to know the patients. Her manner is respectful of the patients. |
| | To $O_2$ – Hi darl! Will you come over here and I will make your bed – Did you want to go to the toilet? | Soft tone is used – the nurse invites response. | |
| | $O_2$ I am suffering – I have pain in my leg – I want to see a doctor | This patient walks easily unassisted to the toilet. | |
| | KITCHEN LADY to $O_4$ I am just going to take your tray away. No, I won't take that (glass). There aren't enough around. | There is no response from the nurse – she continues to make the bed. No eye contact – kitchen lady focuses on the tray. | |

record observed interactions (in our example these are conversations) observed behaviours and your comments.

## ▶ Collecting data: considerations for organizing surveys

You have organized your participants to respond to your questionnaires and now your questionnaires are flowing through a number of sources – either internal health agency mail, reply-paid envelopes or research assistants who are manually collecting them from deposit boxes in clinical areas – so what do you do now?

If you have planned your project thoroughly, you will have several things in place before the questionnaires come in. You will have a coding system where you separate the consent form (if applicable) from questionnaire, give each (person) the same code, and store them separately. In your ethics application you may have promised to do one or two things:

1. De-identify the questionnaires so that they become anonymous, and/or
2. Have a method in place whereby you can, if necessary, refer back to the questionnaires to identify any person in case an adverse event occurs during the research.

Part 3

If you code the individual questionnaires and consent forms with the same code number, make sure they are stored separately, in a locked facility, then your method should address both of the previous issues.

## ▶ Providing feedback about your sample

A flow chart provides a clear understanding of potential participant numbers, those able to be consented and those who participated until completion. Randomized trials are now expected to follow the CONSORT

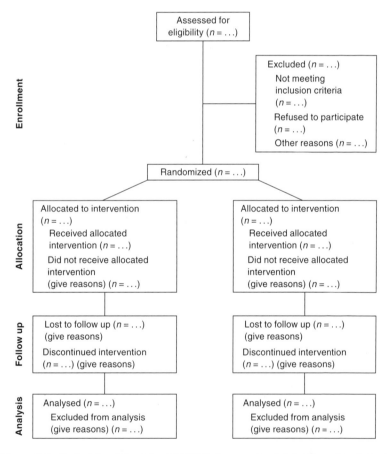

**Figure 7.2** *Revised template of the CONSORT diagram showing the flow of participants through each stage of a randomized trial. (Moher, Schulz and Altman for the CONSORT Group, 2001.)*

Statement as shown in Figure 7.2 (Moher *et al.* 2001) that provides recommendations for presenting results from randomized controlled trials. An example of its application has been presented by Holzhauser *et al.* (2006). Using the flow diagram with the specific components relevant to your method during data collection provides detailed information about the sample in your study.

## ▶ Data entry

### Data entry and analysis responsibilities
Once your data has been collected you need to allocate who is responsible for the following aspects of organizing data to ensure the translation of raw data into data sets does not linger. Using the template below (Figure 7.3) you can create a chart to communicate who is responsible for what task.

### Entry of quantitative data
Now that you have the questionnaires coded and ready to transcribe you need to enter the data into a spreadsheet, statistical database programme, or your chosen way of analysing the results. It is important that your

| Task | Name of responsible officer | Due date |
|---|---|---|
| Developing templates for data entry | | |
| Employing and skilling data entry personnel | | |
| Transcription of interviews or focus group data or observational material | | |
| Data entry into a statistical package or a package for qualitative data | | |
| Decisions on data analysis methods and tests | | |
| Preliminary data analysis (statistical analysis) | | |
| Preliminary thematic analysis of narrative data/transcripts (ideally this is undertaken by a number of members of the team to assist in the cogency of the interpretation) | | |
| Agreement about core constructs and potential areas of exploration | | |
| Feedback of preliminary data analysis to the team | | |
| Decisions about future directions in subsequent analysis (dependant on preliminary findings) | | |
| Report including analysis and preliminary discussion | | |

**Figure 7.3** *Assigning Responsibility*
*(NOTE – Not all these steps will be undertaken for every project. This will depend on the form that the data collection takes)*

Part 3

planning has included decisions about what you are going to use. For quantitative data analysis, one of the most popular and easy to use statistical packages is Statistical Package for Social Sciences (SPSS), which includes its own spreadsheets for data entry. Other computer packages require you to develop your own spreadsheet, while for some, you can enter data into a spreadsheet in Excel, or a database such as Access and then either import them into the statistical package, or perhaps do basic statistics using the functions in those programmes.

## ! Hot Tip: Always check your data entry sheets with the database

Data entry is a job that is best done by the researchers, at least initially, so you know that your spreadsheet or database works the way you expect. Once that is established (and if you have funds), you can hire research assistants and/or clerical staff to input data. Regardless of who is doing this, it is a good idea to check the spreadsheet at intervals. In this way you can check accuracy of entry, and find and rectify mistakes. Even the world's best data entry person is liable to, sometimes, make mistakes. Once you have entered all the data, you should have one of the team check random entries for accuracies. If you are using a package such as SPSS, there are procedures in there for data checking and cleaning. If you are reasonably proficient with such software, you can find these using the help menu; alternatively, buy a book such as the many 'How to . . . ' books readily available, or ask help from someone who regularly uses the package. If you are using software that does not have such facilities, then calculating means and standard deviations or graphs from your data will pick up outliers; in other words, data points which are far larger or smaller than most of the data entered. You can then check if they are real, or if they have resulted from incorrect data entry.

Data entry can be tedious and time-consuming and therefore it is very easy to make errors while entering the data. The data entry checklist below can help you to keep errors to a minimum.

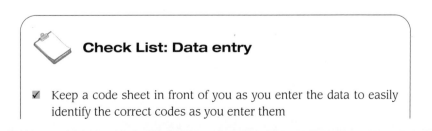

## Check List: Data entry

☑ Keep a code sheet in front of you as you enter the data to easily identify the correct codes as you enter them

☑ Keep a diary to record issues raised during data collection

☑ If there are any changes to data entry coding, ensure this is documented in your diary and on the data code sheet, for example code applied to a response on a Likert scale that falls in between the data points

☑ At the completion of entering your survey, label it numerically so if you identify errors in your entry during the data cleaning process, you can easily identify which survey you need to check.

☑ Be consistent in your coding, for example 'Yes' has the same code assigned throughout the survey.

☑ Press the save button after you have entered each survey.

☑ Backup your data file at the end of each data entry session.

### Creating manageable data from focus groups and interviews

Non-numerical data needs to be made into something manageable that can be analysed. If audio-taped focus groups or interviews have to be transcribed, you must decide if you are going to do it yourself, or if it is to be done by someone else, in which case that person may need to be paid. Other methods, such as note-taking or video-filming, will need just as much organization beforehand to make sure you capture all the richness of the data.

If you are using transcriptions of interviews or other qualitative methods, it is best to check the accuracy of the transcriptions by reading through the transcriptions while listening to the audiotapes. Checking the transcription of data, while often tedious, is a very important part of any research project.

Once tapes, whether from focus groups or interviews, are transcribed, they need to be analysed. Analysis of qualitative data requires reading and re-reading, initially independent analysis should be undertaken. After this, everyone should meet and discuss the interpretation, and justification of interpretation. If a theoretical methodology has been used then this will purposely direct the analysis (Henderson 2005). Alternatively, where the data requires thematic analysis, texts such as Miles and Huberman (1994) provide comprehensive direction in the data analysis process.

Suffice to say that organization of the process to get your data, in whatever form, ready for analysis, is important and cannot be left to chance. If you are unsure about this, ask for help from someone who has done it before. Always remember to thank them (or anyone who helps you) in the acknowledgements passage of the paper or dissertation which is the end result of the research project.

**Part 3**

### Searching archives: using a framework to enter data

Working with archives can be great fun, and walking into a room full of them can be like walking into Aladdin's cave. But like Aladdin, it is often very difficult to know where to start. On your first visit, familiarize yourself with the archive and its data; you will have begun to form ways to collect what you need from it. Keeping your research question in your mind, look for places that will yield the information you need to answer it. Once you are sure such information is there, attend to the following:

- Examine how the records are structured;
- How they are stored;
- What each page or record contains;
- How legible the entries are. (This can be a real headache if using very old records. A researcher examining anti-tobacco lobbying in the 1600s examined broadsheets [the precursors to newspapers] and leaflets of the time, and took three months to learn to read the print and differentiate words where the common usage of the time was to substitute 'f' for 's' in some words.)

Devise a coding system which will allow you to

a) find the record again, and
b) allow you to link your records with the archive, and cross-reference your own records.

It is impossible to give a set format for tools to examine and collect data from archives. However, the checklist below will help you remember several key issues.

## Check List: Key issues when archiving

- ☑ You always need to be able to find the section in the archive where you collected the piece of information
- ☑ You may need to cross-reference what you are finding with your own records, with other parts of the archive, and with existing literature or another set of archives
- ☑ You may have to stop and come back to the work at some later time, so you must have a system that enables you to immediately continue the work without scratching your head and wondering where on earth you were up to

## ▶ Keeping records

It is essential to keep a very good filing system. Ideally, one draw in a filing cabinet or even a whole filing cabinet (depending on the size of the project) can be convenient. The paper continues to mount with the collection of articles, various forms of ethics submissions, handwritten notes of the arrangements that are made at various meetings, followed by copies of the emails sent to the relevant parties confirming the arrangements made at the meetings, and the responses and clarification before approval is given for such things as access, release of staff and so on. Include the tools, surveys/questionnaires, transcribed focus group data and/or interview transcriptions, data sheets and backup of data analysis.

### Keeping track of literature

Keeping a track of records of the research process needs considerable organization. Keep the literature review in an orderly fashion with the continuous collection of articles. If there are too many articles on a particular section, it is useful to categorize them further. Increasingly, articles are being stored in PDF format that saves the large boxes of articles that many of us struggle to keep in alphabetical order! Given this however, there are still many articles that are only available in paper form. In particular, there are seminal papers that we find ourselves constantly re-visiting. It is essential to keep all these articles together for simplicity when we need to access them. The computer program Endnote™ can assist in cataloguing both the paper and PDF format.

---

### ⚠ Hot Tip: Keeping track of the literature

Identify a logical system early in the research process and stick with it to enhance easy retrieval of your literature/documents.

---

### Keeping track of reports and word files

When filing word documents relating to the research, a clear system for version control can be very useful. A strategy to highlight most recent versions is putting the date. Remember that computers store documents in numerical and alphabetical order, so use a numerical system that will place the files in order. However, it is often useful to have 'full draft' or 'shortened draft' in the title of the word document because sometimes the final version is a smaller version of the initial draft. This can be problematic when we want to re-visit the project in a different context and want the broader literature! Make sure word or excel documents are clear and easily identifiable when retrieved so that time is not wasted on finding the exact version of the document when needed.

## Management of difficult situations during data collection

The intention is that data collection will run to plan; however, extraneous events do impact on data collection and these need to be appropriately managed and reported. These may include identification of an illness that requires unplanned intervention for the participants' well being, or even a situation that occurs within the clinical setting that is not related to the research but may affect the data collection process. It is important to have strategies in place or to be flexible to manage these issues as they arise.

## ▶ Summary

This chapter has discussed the practicalities of organizing the team to ensure that the data collection has been undertaken in a systematic fashion. Whether the data be in the form of surveys, tapes, videos, or written notes it needs to be meticulously collected and a system needs to be established to progress the analysis of the data (even if it is an agreed set of meetings with the team). There are particular considerations that are worthwhile remembering for particular methods to ensure rigour in the process. If there is insufficient detail in the data that has been collected then this will directly affect the cogency of the analysis of the data – this will be discussed in Chapter 8.

## ▶ References

Davis, C., Cooke, M., Holzhauser, K., Jones, M. and Finucane, J. (2005). The effect of aromatherapy massage with music on the stress and anxiety levels of emergency nurses. *Australasian Emergency Nursing Journal*, 8(1–2): 43–50.

Fox, R., Henderson, A. and Malko-Nyhart, K. (2006). RESEARCH-IN-BRIEF: A comparison of preceptor and preceptee's perception of how the perceptor role was operationalized. *Journal of Clinical Nursing*, 15: 361–4.

Henderson, A. (2005). The integration of interpretive research approaches: their value in 'capturing' health care context. *Journal of Advanced Nursing*, 52(5): 554–60.

Holzhauser, K., Finucane, J. and De Vries, S.M. (2006) Family Presence During Resuscitation: A randomised controlled trial of the impact of family presence. *Australasian Emergency Nursing Journal* 8(4): 139–47.

Miles, M.B. and Huberman, A.M. (1994). *Qualitative Data Analysis: An Expanded Sourcebook* (2nd edn). Sage Publications, Thousand Oaks, CA.

Moher, D., Schulz, K.F. and Altman, D.G. (2001). 'The CONSORT Statement: Revised Recommendations for Improving the Quality of Reports of Parallel-Group Randomized Trials', The CONSORT Group, viewed 11 September 2006, <http://www.consort-statement.org/Statement/figure1.htm>.

# Chapter eight

# The interpretation and analysis of your findings: gaining value from the research process

*Amanda Henderson and Kerri Holzhauser*

► **Contents**

▷ Organising the data
▷ Examining the data
▷ Reporting meaningful findings
▷ Pointers when reporting
▷ What do you do with your data upon completion

In this chapter we show you how to make sense of the data you have collected and report it correctly. This is not a chapter on analysing data in the statistical sense, rather in keeping with the theme of this book, we present some practical tips on how to manage this process. There are three stages to consider. First, you need to *organize the data* to make interpretation easier; second you need to *examine the data* and decide what aspects are important (implicit in this is identifying the community that the findings have relevance); and finally, you need to *present the data* in a manner that is easily understood and is of interest to those who read it. For those readers who would like to consider how to choose and use an appropriate research method we have provided a further reading guide at the end of this chapter to assist you with this endeavour.

The way you do this will vary depending on whether the data you have collected is qualitative or quantitative. Quantitative data, comprised of numerical values, are analysed using statistical processes and are presented as figures mainly in the form of tables and/or graphs. Alternatively, qualitative data, comprised of narrative statements or images, are organized according to themes or specific forms specified in the methodology. For example, a study that uses conversational analysis will present findings in terms of examples of dialogue. These two different types of data are reported and analysed in different ways and we will discuss these separately.

There is a lot of excellent literature available on data analysis, and you may well want to investigate it further. Their chapter is intended to provide a brief introduction only.

## ▶ Organizing the data

### Quantitative data

Quantitative data is data comprised of numbers. The analysis of quant-itative data requires a good understanding and working knowledge of statistics. It is important that you have someone in your team who has these skills or that you employ a statistician to assist you with calcu-lating your sample size and the data that should be collected. Ideally, you will have addressed this in your *master proposal* including the type of statistical program and a broad overview of the statistical tests you will use.

## ⁞ Hot Tip

If you are employing a statistician, involve them from the beginning of the project. They can advise you about the adequacy of your sample size, realistic numbers of variables and statistical tests appropriate for your data.

The size of the data set and type of data will influence the management and analysis of the data. Developing a data analysis plan can help you to manage the data and to keep track of your analysis. The plan includes your hypotheses or questions and a table describing

- the variable names,
- the measurement level of the data, for example nominal, ordinal, scale or ratio,
- the type of variable, for example dependent or independent, and
- the codes and their values.

A data analysis plan template has been provided below. To use it, place the hypotheses, all the variables, their measurement type and codes in the corresponding rows or columns. Then, looking at your hypotheses, in the intersecting box for the dependent and independent variables, list the statistical tests you will use, for example frequencies, mean, median, *t*-test, correlation, ANOVA and so on. If you have a statistician to undertake the statistical analysis for you then you may want to list the hypotheses, variables and codes. The plan will help you to keep a clear understanding of the data you have and will help decipher the codes when you get your statistical analysis report.

## Data analysis plan

| Hypothesis(es): | | | | | | | |
|---|---|---|---|---|---|---|---|
| | | Dependent variables | | | | | |
| | | Variable | e.g. Sex | | | | Variable Codes |
| Independent variables | Variable | Measurement type | Nominal | | | | |
| | | | | | | | |
| | | | | | | | |
| | | | | | | | |
| | | | | | | | |
| | | | | | | | |
| | | | | | | | |
| | Variable Codes | | 1. Male 2. Female | | | | |

(NOTE: how much of this plan is used will depend on your participation in the data analysis)

## Qualitative data

The narratives and/or expressions derived from qualitative data are not as easily organized as the numerical data derived from quantitative research. In the first instance the data needs to be transcribed or organized into a format that can be more readily analysed; the number and duration of occasions that data were collected; the number and profile of participants; and the setting(s). All this information needs to be organized in a logical fashion so that it can be easily retrieved when required. The demographic information and details of data collection periods can be recorded on simple excel documents; however, organizing the actual data to explore trends, themes and generation of meaning can be logistically complex. How you approach the analysis of the data will be determined by your chosen methodology or the conceptual framework that underpins your work. It is important that the approach and the premise upon which qualitative data is collected is made explicit at the beginning of your work (and this should be clearly explained in the *master proposal*) as this can not be changed 'mid stream' without affecting the rigour of the findings. When you have decided the methodological approach, then the following pointers and programs may assist you in organizing your data. What you use needs to be congruent with your specific approach.

The computer program *Ethnograph*™, first developed in the early 1980s, is a fairly simple database whereby text-based findings can be stored. More recently, *NUD*ST*™ and *NVIVO*™ have been developed. These programs do not really analyse the data but rather sort it according to the structure that you have decided upon. This is called a 'tree diagram'.

In the absence of these better developed systems there is still considerable qualitative analysis undertaken by pen and paper. In qualitative research the researchers become immersed in the data which is usually produced in copious amounts! It is important for the researcher(s) to read, re-read, think and reflect on what is expressed in the qualitative data. Normally, several researchers in the team will do this. During the process of reading and re-reading, it is important to revisit the literature. It is useful to re-visit the 'mind map' or 'concept map' that is often a part of the initial stages of conceptualizing the research prior to the development of the proposal. This can provide a trigger or a reminder of the key factors that were driving the research when it was commenced. As mentioned in Chapter 7, depending on the theoretical approach used in data collection, the data analysis needs to follow the same premise. In preparation for the examination of the data the key ideas/points can be enlarged and put on a board or physically placed on a large table to assist with organizing categories.

## ▶ Examining the data

Now the exciting part has arrived! You, someone in the team or an independent statistician has run the data through statistical analyses and determined significant differences or correlations; or you and the team have explored the written material and identified commonalities and differences that you have grouped. This is where you examine the findings and interpret or make suggestions about what the findings may mean.

### Quantitative data

Thought and consideration needs to be given to why this information was collected in the first place – referring back to the initial questions will assist you to focus and reflect on the findings. Common questions you might ask when you look at the data should be based on the initial objectives/hypotheses of the research. Some examples include:

▷ What are the trends in descriptive statistics? (Descriptive data is most frequently used to analyse populations and samples therefore questions about how representative a population is in relation to the demographic data is useful)

▷ What are the differences in the results? (This may be between samples or demographics)

▷ Has a relationship between two variables been identified? (If there appears to be little of interest between particular groups, it is worth exploring different combinations of groups that you may not have initially considered).

---

## ! Hot Tip: Taking care with interpretations

Do not make interpretations that have no foundation. For example, if you have collected broad occupational data on medical officers and do not specify levels within the occupation (such as specialist medical officer or resident medical officer), you can only interpret the data for the whole occupation not levels within that occupation.

---

Attempt to put the information in perspective. To do this, you relate your results back to the clinical environment. Why are these results significant given the nature context of the work undertaken? What happens within the work environment that may influence the results? Further to interpreting whether a change did or did not occur in response to an intervention, analyse the factors in the environment which may have influenced a positive or negative result such as staffing levels, the nature or extent of an intervention, prevailing motivation/attitudes in the area or specific events/interventions or unprecedented changes in practice.

### Qualitative analysis

With large bundles of paper and extensive descriptions the organization and derivation or creation of meaning is a complex task. Due to the strict processes that justify the rigour of the findings, you need extensive information around how your data was obtained (and in some cases, meanings clarified when it was obtained). Exhaustive findings can also reduce ambiguity in meaning. While this is not always possible or even necessary with some methods, it is important with text-based data that the meanings are well argued. When making sense and justifying the description developed through qualitative analysis, it is acceptable to present the findings and the discussion within the same section of the report/publication. When using this form of presentation, the findings can be discussed in relation to other literature – this assists in strengthening the argument that you are presenting.

## ! Hot Tip: Getting your qualitative findings on to paper

The research team usually discusses the qualitative data as part of the analysis. To make it easier to move the findings to paper, record the research team's discussion and use the discussion as a starting point.

## ▶ Reporting meaningful findings

### Presentation of data

Descriptive statistics can be presented *numerically in tables or graphically*, or *both*. Visual representation in a graph can be powerful. It is important to consider what is most significant – and consider presenting this in some visual form. The form of presentation is usually decided after examining the data and determining the most salient features of the data. Careful and judicious use of visual figures can be compelling when emphasizing a particular point. An example of this is in the Zernike and Henderson study that uses a graph to report on the effectiveness of a constipation risk scale (1999, p. 109). From the graph, it is quite obvious that the risk scale is quite effective for only one risk group.

Inferential statistics identify whether differences in the results are statistically significant thereby they are able to suggest if there is a relationship between different variables. The results of the analysis of variance should be discussed with reference to a table or graph of the group means. Describe the relevant outcomes and back up any claims with the results of statistical tests, however, do not let the statistical analysis become the focus of the discussion. Instead, use statistical analysis to substantiate your findings.

Part 3

## Reporting results

When reporting results, the following general rules should be used as a guide: The results should be presented in plain English; the use of statistical jargon should be limited; and the findings explained so that they can stand on their own. To do this properly, you need to look at the results and identify their importance to the wider professional and/or lay community. The most challenging aspect of reporting research is identifying why it is important. While you may have proved or disproved your hypothesis, the possible reasons for this still needs to be logically argued. If the research did not propose a hypothesis then the team needs to reflect on their initial reason for embarking on the research. The findings need to be considered in view of the question(s) that was asked. Often peripheral information emerges, and this needs to be considered it may to be of significance if it has emerged in the course of your questions.

---

## ! Hot Tip: Dealing with unexpected results

Even if the results are negative, that is your expectations are not forthcoming, it is important to disseminate your findings as this adds to the body of literature in your field and perhaps prevents others taking a similar path.

---

When discussing the results, it is important you relate your results back to the literature. This may mean: comparing your results with the results of others and discuss why they may be different or the same; or how these results will impact/influence practice.

### Putting the information in perspective

Clinical research often involves taking apart different aspects of practices and viewing it in isolation to examine the contribution of a component part (Henderson 2006). If this is the situation with your particular study then it is essential that the discussion of the study revisits the whole picture. This will clarify the significance of the project and assist in giving the research meaning. Examining the data to identify its importance to the wider professional and/or lay community is essential. While you may have proved or disproved your hypothesis, the possible reasons and significance of this still needs to be logically argued.

## Issues with reporting findings

When undertaking research, the results are not always as expected. This was the case with a study exploring how registered nurses designated as 'preceptors' supported new graduates. In this project an unexpected finding revealed that registered nurses were often not available to precept the new graduate. Instead, new graduates who transitioned to the work place successfully identified their own support person (Fox *et al.* 2006). Although this was not the expected finding, it is still worth disseminating.

It is essential that you recognize and address limitations in your research process. For example, was the process appropriate to answer the questions you wanted answered?

## What to do with your data when the project is completed

Data needs to be stored in a secure locality for quite a long period of time following completion. This varies between countries, facilities and types of data. Most facilities have a policy on this so make sure that you check yours and adhere to the requirements.

## ▶ Summary

At the completion of the collection and compilation of the data, the process of making sense of what it means can almost seem daunting. It is important that you have considered how you will undertake this task from the beginning, as assumptions made at the outset will influence the data analysis. This chapter provides some pointers on how you can organize this data ready for the process you have decided for analysis. In addition, suggestions have been made to revisit the initial questions, and also conceptual maps that were developed when you were proposing the research. This can be a useful guide during the interpretation of your research, where you need to explain to the wider community why it was important that your research was conducted.

## ▶ References

Fox, R., Henderson, A. and Malko, K. (2006). Research-in-brief: A comparison of preceptor and preceptee's perception of how the preceptor role was operationalised. *Journal of Clinical Nursing*, 15: 361–4.

Part 3

Henderson, A. (2006). Guest editorial – 'maximising value from clinical research'. *Journal of Clinical Nursing*, 15(12): 147.

Zernike, W. and Henderson, A. (1999). Evaluation of a constipation risk scale. *International Journal of Nursing Practice*, 5(2): 106–9.

## ▶ Further reading for guidance on the application of research methods

This chapter has provided an overview of the practical considerations on how to manage the data analysis process. It has not provided any detail on research methods or methodology. In the following list we provide a number of texts that we use and refer to regularly in our own work.

De Vaus David (2001). *Research Design in Social Research*. Sage, London.

▷ This is one of our favourites because it focuses on research design in a clear and concise manner. Issues covered include testing theories, causation, data analysis and the main considerations involved in using the different research designs.

Greene, J.C. and Caracelli, V.J. (1997). *Advances in Mixed-Method Evaluation: The Challenges and Benefits of Integrating Diverse Paradigms*. Jossey-Bass Publishers, San Francisco.

▷ This text provides a great overview of the types of mixed-methods and some examples of applying mixed-method research. It is very easy to read and understand.

Miles, M.B. and Huberman, A.M. (1994). *Qualitative Data Analysis: An Expanded Sourcebook* (2nd edn). Sage Publications, Thousand Oaks, CA.

▷ This book provides comprehensive and practical methods of analysing qualitative data. It outlines the issues of qualitative data analysis and practical information on illustrating the analysis, variations and advice to make the analysis process easier.

Minichiello, V., Sullivan, G., Greenwood, K. and Axford, R. (eds) (2003). *Handbook of Research Methods for Nursing & Health Science* (2nd edn). Prentice Hall Health, Frenchs Forest, NSW.

▷ This book provides researchers in health care with a broad overview of a variety of research methods. It is comprehensive, user-friendly and an excellent resource for embarking on the research process.

Parahoo, K. (2006). *Nursing Research: Principles, Process and Issues*. Palgrave Macmillan, Basingstoke, England.

▷ This is another one of our favourites because it is so comprehensive yet easy to follow. This edition also features new chapters on qualitative research, quantitative research, combining qualitative and quantitative methods and evidence-based practice, and there are expanded sections on research governance, systematic reviews and the utilization of research.

Polit, D.F. and Beck, C.T. (2006). *Essentials of Nursing Research: Methods, Appraisal, and Utilisation* (6th edn). Lippincott Williams & Williams, Philadelphia.

▷ This is a well-known and comprehensive text that provides an introductory overview of multiple qualitative and quantitative research methods.

Tabachnick, B.G. and Fidell, L.S. (2007). *Using Multivariate Statistics* (5th edn) Pearson/Allyn & Bacon, Boston.

▷ This text provides a more advanced but easy to understand practical overview of common statistical and multivariate analysis techniques. It provides description and syntax examples for applying these tests in a variety of statistical analysis programmes, for example SPSS, SAS.

# Chapter nine

# Disseminating findings

*Sarah Winch*

## ▶ Contents

- ▷ Unit-based education meetings
- ▷ Grand rounds (discipline specific or interdisciplinary)
- ▷ Poster presentations at conferences
- ▷ Conference papers
- ▷ Panel presentations
- ▷ Research reports
- ▷ Published abstracts
- ▷ Journal articles
- ▷ Book chapters
- ▷ Newspapers – press releases and feature articles

In this chapter we present a number of different ways to present research findings and disseminate new knowledge to a variety of audiences. Many clinical professions tend to pass on knowledge through stories at 'handover', during practice and through observation. While in the past this may have served them well, in the current climate it is vital for these professions to articulate, measure, review and communicate the role they have in modern health care. In this way they have the tools and evidence to value and justify their position in the healthcare budget.

Despite this imperative, many clinicians find this the most challenging aspect of research work. In our experience, clinical staff are happy to be involved in the conduct of research by deriving a question and collecting data but much less keen on writing literature reviews, journal and newspaper articles or books. This makes the publication of research findings a daunting prospect. Sharing this task with more experienced writers can help newer researchers and clinical partners to overcome some of their hesitation.

While most research should result in a publication, this is not always the case. Many clinicians increase their knowledge by attending study days or short conferences where they can update their skills on technology and care practices. For the researcher this is an important factor to consider when considering where and how to disseminate their results for the best effect. In the following check list we identify some of the most useful ways to disseminate your research.

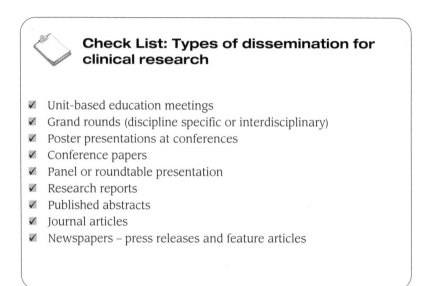

**Check List: Types of dissemination for clinical research**

☑ Unit-based education meetings
☑ Grand rounds (discipline specific or interdisciplinary)
☑ Poster presentations at conferences
☑ Conference papers
☑ Panel or roundtable presentation
☑ Research reports
☑ Published abstracts
☑ Journal articles
☑ Newspapers – press releases and feature articles

## ▶ Choosing how to disseminate research

Depending on the outcome that you seek there are a myriad of ways and places to disseminate your findings. The best way to decide where you should start is to consider your audience. Table 9.1 can help you to decide.

**Table 9.1** *Disseminating findings*

| Target audience | Type of material | Disseminating mode |
|---|---|---|
| Practising clinicians | Clinical practice measurement, review and evaluation | Unit meetings Grand rounds Clinical conferences |
| Health academics | Clinical practice innovation Case studies with a focus on theory or method The development of clinical practice models Large scale research studies | Practice journals University seminar series Broad-based clinical conferences Academic journals |
| Policy makers | Impacts of health, clinical or welfare policy on patients or the healthcare system | Academic journals Industry reports Government reports |

Part 3

**Table 9.1**   *(Continued)*

| Target audience | Type of material | Disseminating mode |
|---|---|---|
| Health disciplines (medicine, social work, nursing, physiotherapy, occupational therapy) | Broad-based patient safety and health worker issues | Interdisciplinary practice journals |
| Other disciplines (ethics, law, education, business, sociology psychology) | Any material that uses a clinical focus in any of these discipline areas. For example, the effects of shift work on clinicians. | Interdisciplinary practice journals |

## Unit-based education meetings

These meetings are usually convened at regular intervals throughout the year to update all staff and keep them clinically relevant. You can use these meetings as a communication tool throughout your entire project. It makes sense to present your initial ideas here, to gain broad-based support and then to keep staff abreast of (and interested in) your project throughout the time it takes to complete. This is a great place to practice to a reasonably friendly audience and refine your presentation.

Although this is a local audience, you should treat this opportunity to present seriously. Prepare as you would for a conference presentation. 'PowerPoint™', part of the Microsoft office suite of computer programs, is an excellent presentation tool that is easy to learn. You will need access to the program and audiovisual equipment such as a data projector to show your PowerPoint™. If you are unable to get access to audiovisual equipment then prepare using the PowerPoint™ format and print them out using the 'handouts' choice in the print selection. This will give you practice at preparing PowerPoint™ and give the audience some visual cues to follow. While PowerPoint™ is becoming one of the most common forms of presentation, it can be used poorly. Use the following check list to ensure that you are not caught out overloading your audience!

### Check List: Avoiding 'death by PowerPoint™'

- ☑ Consider you audience and time frame
- ☑ Don't have too many slides; less is best
- ☑ Don't use lengthy quotes
- ☑ Don't include a lengthy literature review

- ☑ Don't get carried away by some of the audio features; they can be distracting
- ☑ Summarize key points and arguments
- ☑ Talk separately about examples
- ☑ Include data: this is a great way to summarize
- ☑ Select the best images and check copyright!
- ☑ Avoid reading your slides
- ☑ Maintain eye contact with your audience

### Grand rounds

Grand rounds have a long history in medical training and are now becoming more common in other health professions. These educational meetings are held regularly in facilities to update colleagues on new protocols and procedures for patient care, or to discuss unusual case studies and present research results. This type of meeting provides an opportunity to present to a wider, perhaps multidisciplinary audience. Again, you need to treat this event seriously and put in the same careful preparation in terms of content and presentation as a conference. Check the likely professional background of your audience. For example, do medical or nursing staff predominate? Note the length of time you have to present and the time for audience questions.

### Poster presentations at conferences

Many conferences welcome the submission of posters for inclusion in their program. These involve a visual presentation of the beginning stage or the results from a research project. Guidelines from the conference organisers will be issued on the size of the posters and it is important to adhere to these as there is often limited space for poster display.

### ⁝ Hot Tip: Covering the costs of posters

Posters can be expensive to make and are a legitimate cost in a grant application. Check whether your facility has a graphic art or medical illustration department. Frequently, these can help you produce a professional poster for a reduced fee.

Part 3

Posters can be displayed for the length of the conference or for a single day. You may be asked to talk about your poster or stand by it and answer questions in the poster viewing times during the conference. If you have the resources, handouts explaining the poster more fully can be placed nearby. The following check list provides a general guide for what posters should contain.

---

### Check List: Inclusions for a great poster

☑ The name of your study
☑ All of the research team's names
☑ The ethics approval number
☑ Your hypothesis, research question or area
☑ An outline of your findings best displayed as charts, graphs or, perhaps, photographs
☑ Acknowledgements of your funding body and clinical supporters

---

## Conference papers

Conference presentations are a great way of presenting your findings and receiving some constructive feedback on your work. Writing a conference presentation is a good motivator prior to proceeding with the paper to publication. Before you start working on your presentation, you need to choose an appropriate conference that will showcase your work. Not all conference papers are the same and will vary from discipline to discipline; for example in the humanities and social sciences it is not uncommon for presenters to read their paper without any visual aids. If your work has the potential to be presented at an interdisciplinary conference, make sure that you are aware of the preferred mode of presentation. If you are attending the entire conference (always a good idea when you are presenting), you can get a feel for the audience and the type of questions asked. Some questions may be critical of your topic, method, findings or all of these things. Before you deliver your paper, ask a friend to read it who will give you a honest feedback. Practice answering difficult or critical questions. Make sure you understand your time limit and stick to it even if other presenters are not as disciplined! This should allow for questions and you will get valuable feedback for your work. Prepare your presentation using the following check list.

---

### Check List: Developing a conference presentation

☑ Decide on authors, order of the authors and acknowledgements.

☑ Decide on who will present. This person should become the team leader and take responsibility for submission to the conference and producing the final product.

☑ Identify the 'hook and the heart' of your presentation. Why would people come and listen to it?

☑ Write a working title.

☑ Make sure this fits in with the conference that you are targeting.

☑ Familiarize yourself with the conference requirements (type and length of papers).

☑ Identify the main sections (problems, methods, data, discussion and recommendations).

☑ Allocate the main sections to the authors and allow them one slide for each section!

☑ Write timelines in accordance with the conference submission deadlines.

☑ Assemble the first draft and review all the tables and figures.

☑ Check to see if there are some suitable pictures that you can use.

☑ Circulate the second draft to all authors for reading and editing.

☑ Confirm the title.

☑ Write the abstract.

☑ Submit the abstract to the conference organizers.

---

### Panel or roundtable presentation

Panel sessions usually include a small group of speakers that each present or respond to questions on a particular issue or theme. A chairperson manages the flow of questions and directs them to each panel member. Panelists are usually invited to take part as recognition of their expertise. To prepare as a panelist, you need to know the professional background of your audience and their knowledge of your field. Ask what your involvement will be. Are you to respond to questions or give a short presentation and then respond to questions? Once again, take care to stick to your time limit.

### Writing abstracts

An abstract is a summary of your paper that overviews your question, method and results in a very concise format. Abstracts are required for conference and journal paper submissions. They are not always easy to write and are often best left until you have finished your paper or presentation completely. Some journals and conferences prefer a structured abstract like the following written by Sarah Winch, Amanda Henderson and Debra Creedy (2005) and published in the *Journal of Advanced Nursing* (see Figure 9.1). For this theoretical paper the authors have structured the abstract according to the guidelines by clearly identifying the aim, background and discussion in a structured manner that makes it easy for the reader to follow.

In the following example (Figure 9.2) a similar format has been used for a research paper.

Winch, S., Henderson, A., and Creedy, D. (2005)

Read, Think, Do!: a method for fitting research evidence into practice

Aim. This paper discusses a process for research utilization that overcomes well known barriers in order to influence clinical decision-making and practice change. Read, Think, Do! is a problem-solving approach to research utilization and practice development which has the potential to overcome barriers to research utilization.

Background. Any process for research utilization at the practice level needs to overcome numerous barriers in order to influence clinical decision-making and practice change. Access to research-based knowledge is an obvious first step in the evidence-based approach to care delivery, but is clearly inadequate alone in influencing the improvement of practice.

Discussion. Read, Think, Do! acknowledges the complexity of problem-solving processes from the outset by looking for (1) the evidence, (2) assessing the value to practice, and (3) addressing the social and cultural milieu of the practice setting to ascertain the best strategies for initiating and sustaining practice change. This approach draws distal forms of empirical knowledge that have the capacity to improve patient outcomes into the proximal knowledge base of the clinical nurse. This is achieved by collaboration, planning and evaluation involving all levels of staff and a specialist facilitator, the Clinical Nurse Consultant in evidence-based practice.

Conclusion. Read, Think, Do! is a method of research utilization and practice development that has the potential to overcome barriers to research utilization and avoid the 'misplaced concreteness' that can occur when trying to fit empiricism into practice. By addressing the breadth and diversity of issues surrounding research utilization in a systematic manner it presents a sustainable method for practice change informed by evidence.

Keywords: research utilization, nursing, evidence-based practice

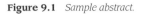

**Figure 9.1** *Sample abstract.*

Henderson, A., Winch, S., Holzhauser, K. and DeVries, S. (2006)

The motivation of health professionals to explore research evidence in their practice: An intervention study

Aim: To assess the impact of multifaceted clinically focused educational strategies that concentrated on introducing dementia care research evidence on health professionals' awareness and inclination to use research findings in their future practice.

Background: The promise of evidence-based practice is slow to materialise with the limitations of adopting research findings in practice readily identifiable.
Method: A pre- and post-test quasi experimental design. The study involved: the administration of a research utilisation survey as a pre-test (baseline); an intervention phase; and a post-test survey, the same research utilisation survey.

Tool: The Edmonton Research Orientation Survey (EROS), a self-report tool that asks participants about their attitudes toward research and about their potential to use research findings, was used to determine to health professionals orientation to research.

Intervention: The introduction of dementia care research evidence through multi-faceted clinically focused educational strategies to improve practice. This was achieved through a resource team comprising: a Clinical Nurse Consultant, as a leader and resource of localised evidence-based knowledge in aged care; an experienced registered nurse to support the introduction of strategies and a further experienced educator and clinician to reinforce the importance of evidence in change.

Results: Across all the four subscales that are measured in the EROS survey, statistical analysis by independent samples t-test identified that there was no significant change between the before and after measurements.

Relevance to clinical practice: Successful integration of changes based on evidence does not necessarily mean that staff become more aware or are more inclined to use research findings in the future to address problems.

Key words: evidence, research practice, intervention, dementia care

**Figure 9.2** *Sample research paper abstract.*

Note also the use of key words. These are an important part of the article because they will identify your work to others working on your field when they search using an electronic information retrieval system.

### Check List: Writing abstracts

☑ Identify the requirements as specified by the publisher or conference organizer such as word length. Most abstracts are approximately 150–250 words in length.

**Check List (Continued)**

☑ Reread your research findings.

☑ Identify the hook and the heart for your paper.

☑ Outline in draft the purpose, methods, scope, results, conclusions and recommendations.

☑ Try to avoid copying sentences from your paper, and summarize in a new way.

☑ Polish your draft so that it reads well and has no errors.

## ▶ Writing journal articles

Having presented your paper at a conference, unit meeting or grand rounds, taken on board some good feedback or criticism, it is time to progress the paper to a journal publication. Many academic journals have websites that tell you the sort of material that they like to publish and provide specific instructions for authors. Obviously, the *Journal of Paediatrics* will not be interested in your work on nutrition in patients with Alzheimer's disease. However, some other choices are less clear-cut. Some journals focus on publishing particular methods or theoretical approaches. If it is not clear where to submit your article from the information on the journal website then read several of the journals themselves. This will give you an accurate idea of the work that they are publishing.

### The role of 'impact factors'

An impact factor is a way of measuring the importance of academic journals and the papers they contain. An impact factor measures the frequency that the 'average article' in a journal has been cited in a particular year or period. Important scientific journals such as *Nature* have high impact factors. Many healthcare journals do not have an impact factor at all. If you are trying to build your track record, then you should select the most appropriate journal with the highest impact factor. Research funders view this as a mark of quality of the journal. If you want to influence practice in a particular field that has a journal that is read widely by clinical staff but has a low impact factor, then this should also be a consideration.

### Use of style guides and Endnote™

The journal that you submit will specify the style that you must use for referencing. This may differ from journal to journal. The information for authors should specify the referencing and bibliographic style that the journal uses. It is important that you follow what the journal requests. They usually include a list of examples of how they want the reference list and in text references to appear. Read these and follow them carefully. If no examples are provided but a style is recommended that you are not familiar with, the computer software program endnote can help you in this regard. If you do not have this program then borrow or purchase a style guide to assist you or print out the style guide examples given on the journal website. If no style is recommended at all, then use the one that you are familiar with consistently through the paper.

### Writing a good journal article

Writing is a skill that takes practice and discipline. One of the best ways to start is to write with a team with each author taking responsibility for different sections of the paper. The following check list will guide you through the writing process.

## Check List: The writing process

☑ Decide on authors, order of the authors and acknowledgements. Generally, the first author takes responsibility for most of the manuscript including organizing the other authors and corresponding with the publisher.

☑ As a group decide on the hook and the heart for this paper. What is its point of difference from what is already published in this area.

☑ Write a working title.

☑ Identify the correct journal that will best target your audience.

☑ Familiarize yourself with the journal's instructions to authors. These are the requirements specified by the publisher and editors of the journal (length, font, etc.).

☑ Name the main sections (literature review, problem, methods, data collection, discussion and recommendations) and allocate a section or group of sections to each author.

☑ Assemble the first draft.

☑ Review tables and figures.

☑ Prepare any illustrations in the format required by the publisher.

**Check List (Continued)**

☑ Circulate the second draft to all authors for reading and editing.
☑ Rewrite the title.
☑ Write the abstract.
☑ Recheck the instructions for authors and make sure you have complied.
☑ Submit the article to the journal.
☑ Analyse the reviewer's comments and respond appropriately.

After you have the submitted your paper, it will be sent out to several reviewers who will comment on whether the article should be accepted for publication. Their comments will be returned to the submitting author. You are likely to receive one of the following responses:

1. Accept as is with no changes or revisions.
2. Accept the paper once specific changes have been made.
3. Rewrite a substantial proportion of the paper to improve the focus or clarity and then resubmit.
4. Reject.

## Hot Tip: Dealing with unfavourable reviews

You need to develop the hide of an elephant when you begin publishing your work. Most often reviewers will offer very constructive comments. Remember, they publish too! Take these on board and revise your paper. However, if you do receive an unflattering review, which is not constructive, ignore it and submit your paper to another journal.

## ► Research reports

Organizations that fund research often require a report on the progress of the research and at the conclusion of the project that details the findings. It is also a good idea to make a copy of the report for the organization where the research has been conducted. Most funders of research will have a format for you to follow. If they do not provide any, and smaller funding organizations may not, then use the following check list to structure your report. The Chief Investigator needs to take responsibility for completing the research report. Assigning each team member a section to write spreads the work load.

---

**Check List: Sections required for writing a research report**

☑ Title page
☑ Contents
☑ Executive summary (one page only)
☑ Literature review
☑ Methods
☑ Findings
☑ Summary
☑ Recommendations
☑ Appendices (include a verified financial statement on how you have spent the money)

---

Administrators may prefer to read data presented in graph form rather than in tables. This is because it is easy to read and comprehend the data to be presented is complex, think about how you can make the data read easily, using plain language, so that the findings are easily understood.

## ▶ Newspapers: feature articles and press releases

Clinicians rarely write for newspapers or consider them when trying to get important messages or research findings out to the general public. This is an oversight on the part of the clinical professions as a good newspaper article or press release can reach a very large readership quickly and promote their work to the community.

If the message that you are trying to publicize involves the organization that you work for, or a few organizations, it is important to have your work checked before it is submitted to the local newspaper. Many facilities employ public relations officers who are often trained journalists and can help you with this type of writing.

Newspaper articles are short and require a different style of writing from what is used when writing a research report or journal article. Journalists are taught to write in the inverted triangle style ∇ with all the important information given at the start of the first paragraph, working through to specifics at the end.

### Check List: Writing a newspaper article

☑ Check with your facility: Do they have a public relations officer who can help you?
☑ Select an appropriate newspaper to target and make contact with the editor to see if your research fits.
☑ Write an attention-getting headline.
☑ Write your by-line (your name as you wrote the story).
☑ Construct the lead paragraph, this has the most important information (who, what, when, where, why and how).
☑ Add an explanatory paragraph.
☑ Additional information can be in the last paragraph.

Research funders often like to publicize their work. If you hear you are successful in a grant round, prepare a press release to give to the funding organization that they can use.

Princess Alexandra Hospital's Director of Nursing research, Dr Sarah Winch last night received a Queensland Nursing Council (QNC) grant which will fund a significant study into the moral and ethical decisions faced by clinicians in order to develop support systems to retain staff as Queensland faces a nursing shortage.

Hosted by the Queen Elizabeth II Jubilee Hospital, the pilot study is the first part of an Australian component of an international study seeking to measure how clinicians experience, process and resolve ethical dilemmas.

Dr Winch believes these stressful situations may be a contributing factor to why so many clinicians are leaving the profession.

'It is important that we explore the moral and ethical situations many clinicians face in order to gain a better understanding of how we can support them through that process' she said.

'The ability to provide better support to these clinicians would greatly aid recruitment and retention of nursing staff throughout Queensland'.

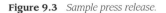

**Figure 9.3** *Sample press release.*

An example of a press release has been supplied as Figure 9.3. This was written by Sarah Winch on the request of the funders, the Queensland Nursing Council who wanted to publicize their 2006 grant round.

## ▶ Summary

Taking the next step to publish your findings is often a difficult one but it is critical to the accumulation of the evidence base of the health professions. The chief investigator plays a key role in this process and should always ensure that findings are disseminated in whatever is the most appropriate manner for the stage of the research. For example, it is perfectly acceptable for 'work in progress' to be presented as conference papers or posters. To balance the load of writing reports and publications, ensure that all team members take a part in the process. Now that you have taken the time and effort to truly ground your work in the clinical setting and produce findings that are useful and relevant to clinical practice – we all need to hear about it!

## ▶ References

Henderson, A., Winch, S., Holzhauser, K. and DeVries, S. (2006). The motivation of health professionals to explore research evidence in their practice: an intervention study. *Journal of Clinical Nursing*, 15(12): 1559–64.

Winch, S., Henderson, A. and Creedy, D. (2005). Read Think Do! fitting empiricism into practice. *Journal of Advanced Nursing*, April, 50(1): 20–6.

# Chapter ten

# Creating and sustaining research-friendly environments

*Sarah Winch*

## ▶ Contents

▷ Setting the research agenda
▷ Creating research infrastructure
▷ Building research capacity
▷ Research governance and policy: managing the risk associated with research
▷ Measures of success: research performance indicators

Increasingly, healthcare facilities are being asked to determine and shape their research efforts and capabilities. This is not always an easy task given that their key priority is service provision. For those that persevere, the rewards are well worth the effort, with health professionals gaining valuable research expertise and knowledge that emerges directly from the clinical milieux. In this chapter we provide advice for healthcare executives and managers on how to shape their research agenda, build research infrastructure and capacity, and manage the risks associated with these activities.

## ▶ Setting the research agenda: writing the strategic research plan

Health facility executives play a key role in promoting research and setting the research agenda. They are not expected to have the skills to conduct the research (although some may have) but they should be able to set the research direction for the facility and plan how to achieve this. In many ways this is not as difficult as it would seem. Senior healthcare managers use strategic planning regularly to establish the direction of their facility and evaluate performance. The application of these processes to research endeavours is no different.

A strategic research plan should detail the overall direction that you want research to take in your facility or organizational unit. Specific goals, activities, costs and expected results can then be planned out across a reasonable time frame. Start by outlining what you expect to achieve from your research program in broad terms. This will form your overall statement on how you value research at your facility or unit. For example, you may wish to state that you expect the research conducted at your facility to be 'world class', rigorous, objective, ethical, focused on the needs of patients and/or staff and provided in a cost effective, timely and useful manner.

The next step is to detail the key research themes you wish to pursue. Ideally, this should mirror the case-mix of your facility. In this way your research program is integrated with service delivery and can produce useful findings that will assist you with your core business. What you are trying to avoid is a scattering of research effort across the organization that does not produce reliable and meaningful data that you or the wider community can use. This is not to say that small projects should be avoided as they can provide experiential research training for clinical staff in an area of interest to them (as we discuss later in the chapter).

A useful way to start thinking about what direction you should take is to consider the different types of research. The Australian Bureau of Statistics (1998) uses a four type system of activity: pure basic research (medical science laboratory work); strategic basic research; applied research (clinical practice fits here) and experimental development. A more practical way of looking at your future research direction that can potentially optimize outcomes is to consider a balanced mix of problem-driven and core research. Problem-driven research addresses a specific, identified need in order to support an area of clinical practice or healthcare organization. Core research should focus on the key aspects of healthcare delivery including broad areas such as the biological, psycho-social or economic processes that underpin the delivery of health care. Workforce research on recruitment and retention of healthcare staff would fit into this category. These two areas do not need to progress independently. If carefully considered, core research may inform applied research; for example, particular psychological or sociological factors that impact on your facility in a specific way. The following flowchart demonstrates the steps in research planning.

**Part 3**

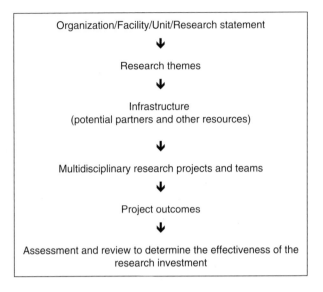

Figure 10.1 *Flow chart for planning research.*

Once your themes are identified, it is possible to organize and prioritize research projects and activities according to these themes. The research team then become the operational unit that is responsible for the progress of the project against agreed milestones. Resources for this team, human and otherwise, can then be determined and allocated. An important part of developing research infrastructure is to establish strategic partnerships with external consultants, tertiary partners or other health facilities to help you achieve the outcomes that are needed. These can assist with a myriad of functions associated with the conduct of research including the application for grant money from external sources.

In the first instance, it is a good idea for the strategic research plan to extend over a three- to five-year period. This time span will allow you to build the infrastructure that you need and to work in alignment with major grant round cycles. Many of the larger grants (which are desirable to access because of the monetary support) extend over a period of three to five years. This is because serious funders of research realize the time factor involved in producing good outcomes. Research projects can be prioritized according to the need, risk, cost and expected benefits of the research to the facility. Where applicable, the research project should include appropriate plans on how the work is to be translated into practice (be that clinical or commercial). This helps the full potential to be realized as findings are incorporated into practice.

## ▶ Communicating and adhering to your research direction

Once you have decided your direction and completed your strategic research plan, you have a framework to communicate with tertiary partners, external commercial entities, collaborators from the other health services and future employees, particularly those at the executive level. Senior management roles are very demanding and can be subject to change when a key figure leaves or when the organization is restructured. If your research direction has been determined, this can reduce some of the instability that follows change at the Executive level. It is important that incoming Executives are aware of the research direction and are willing to provide support for the tenure of the plan. Remember, the production of quality research takes time and changing direction midstream is not helpful as you will lose the time you have spent developing one area and will take additional time to develop another. The risk in changing direction frequently (e.g., with new Executive staff) is that nothing substantial in terms of research is achieved and the initial investment (both in money and goodwill from partners) is lost.

## ▶ Creating research infrastructure

Depending on the direction of your research and the resources that can be drawn upon from partners, your requirements as the service provider may not be that onerous. Social science–based research does not generally require a great deal of support other than office space and associated computer support. If your facility direction is in scientific, biological research then your needs most likely will be different and possibly very expensive. Specialist laboratories for research are costs that are often met through large capital grants provided by governments. This type of support is usually hotly contested and requires long-term specialist planning (and previous indication of success in the area) that is beyond the scope of this chapter.

The following checklist provides an overview of some on the infrastructure needs that a healthcare facility may be able to offer to support research efforts. Many of these are already part of the suite of modern healthcare management services. Other less tangible supports that the organization provides include promoting the research to maximize interest and co-operation and facilitating timely access to the organization and its processes.

**Part 3**

## Check List: Research infrastructure

☑ Dedicated positions to establish and co-ordinate strategic research partnerships or to conduct research and/or allocation of this areas as an Executive portfolio.

☑ Data management – access to statistical and non-numerical data analysis computer programs

☑ Data storage – web space

☑ Information technology support

☑ Office space and equipment

☑ Marketing services and media liaison

☑ Administrative support

☑ Library services

☑ Legal services for oversight of research contracts, protection of intellectual property and assistance with patents

☑ Graphic design and publishing assistance for diagrams, posters and high-quality finishing of research reports and monographs

☑ Finance and human resources: job descriptions, position levels, budget oversight and calculation, establishment of research cost centres

☑ Laboratory space (if funds permit)

If your facility is lacking in any type of research infrastructure then the first goal of your research plan should be to 'Build the infrastructure to support leading-edge research.' An initial step in this process is to recognize this as a specialist area of endeavour and create a senior project officer or assign this area as a portfolio to an executive with research training or expertise.

## ▶ Building research capacity

Increasing an organization's research capacity needs to proceed across two areas. First, the creation of strong research teams with partners that have the capacity to address the research questions generated by the facility (and attract funding) in a sufficiently rigorous manner to provide useful findings. Second, providing opportunities for staff to undertake training in research methods and processes.

Larger facilities may be in the fortunate situation to have resources to dedicate to the growth of research by creating research-specific positions. These range from positions that are funded wholly by the health service such as a Director of Research or Nurse Researcher to those that are jointly funded such as Clinical Chairs or conjoint Lectureships. While the role of these positions may vary, it is critical that a senior officer in the organization takes on the responsibility to create strategic partnerships that promote collaboration and exchange. Where possible, these partnerships should be across disciplines. This way the health service is able to share in expertise outside of its current arena. For example, academics skilled in the emerging discipline of 'Human Factors' examine the interaction between people and the technology they use, can contribute to health care safety and productivity in high technology areas such as Intensive Care Units.

Those facilities that do not have the funds to support dedicated research positions can still attract good academics to work with their clinical staff through the introduction of a Visiting Scholar program. The key is establishing a win-win situation where academics are willing to invest time to get an outcome that will advance their knowledge base and perhaps their career at the same time! Meanwhile, the healthcare facility gains access to years of research training and, depending on the institution that employs the academic, research infrastructure support in terms of an Office of Research and a Research Ethics Committee. For small, isolated facilities that are unable to convene their own research ethics committees these are key resources in progressing their research agenda.

## Making and sustaining contact with local academics

To create a sustainable partnership between academics and clinicians, the research needs to have clinical relevance at an administrative and unit level to ensure involvement, yet still provide a platform for academic success. Care needs to be taken to ensure the research does not become a mechanism for the university to obtain funds for subsequent research that is not useful in the broader sense. An example of this would be a quick small pilot study conducted in a unit that does not have any wider applicability. This is happening more frequently as funding bodies expect pilot studies to have been conducted and published by the researcher before awarding funds. In this case the institution may be asked to pilot a data collection instrument that has no real benefit for the organization long term. They comply but because the instrument is

Part 3

being piloted there is no great value in the findings for that organization. The value may come some years later when the researcher shares findings from a wider study but this can literally take years by which time many of the senior people in the organization have left and no-one can even remember the beginning study! Alternatively, problems may occur if the clinicians 'take over' and ignore expert advice about sound research processes, jeopardizing the rigour and subsequent value of the findings.

## ▶ The 'Visiting Scholar' program

Inviting academics to work with staff requires a policy framework that supports this interaction. Increasing legislation regarding privacy and professional responsibility means that clear parameters need to be set about how this partnership is to proceed. It is critical with these arrangements to ensure that both parties have equal representation, direction and input. Some larger facilities have formal guidelines that set out the parameters for such interaction and these should be included in an appointment letter. Other facilities may wish to enter formal service agreements with the tertiary sector; however, these can become cumbersome and difficult to progress at a local level.

Creating a 'Visiting Scholar' program is a viable alternative that allows clinicians and academics to work together with minimal risk to the organization. A 'Visiting Scholar' program is a cost neutral formal means of originating and producing clinical research via research teams that mix clinicians and academics. Participants from a variety of disciplines are added to strengthen projects as needed. This type of program helps clinicians drive the production of knowledge by raising pertinent clinical questions while the academics provide the methodological rigour to make the project a success.

The program needs to be managed and evaluated by a senior officer within the healthcare facility. This may be the Director of Nursing, or of Clinical Services. It is the responsibility of this person to appoint, monitor and evaluate the scholar's work within the facility. The letter of appointment establishes the conditions by which the facility and the scholar will abide. Each scholar is appointed for a set period and reappointed following a satisfactory review. Key inclusions for the letter are listed in the following check list.

## Check List: Statements to be included in the Visiting Scholar letter of agreement

☑ The amount of time the visiting scholar will be available on site at the facility.

☑ The expectation that the scholar will involve facility staff in the research.

☑ The expectation that the scholar will provide support and guidance according to their particular area of expertise be that methodological or clinical.

☑ The scholar will engage in active involvement, supervision or publication of at least 2 projects per year.

☑ Each scholar will be encouraged to establish his or her own publication collective that involves clinicians.

☑ A list of what the facility will provide such as parking, office space and library facilities, and orientation to the facility's policies and procedures.

☑ A statement affirming the employment status of the scholar such as 'the scholar does not become a member of the facility staff and as such is not to engage in the delivery of nursing care in any situation whilst on site or in any decision-making'.

☑ A statement on the costs involved such as 'This scheme is cost neutral to both parties and as such the scholar will not receive a wage.'

☑ A governance statement relating to research ethics such as 'Scholars must abide by the National Health and Medical Research Council guidelines for research involving human experimentation.'

☑ A governance statement relating to research in the facility such as 'The Scholar must submit all projects to the facility Research Register.'

A Visiting Scholar program should provide benefits for both the academics and clinicians. The academics get access to a patient population and the clinicians to years of research training that the academics have completed!

### ▶ Research training

The facility research plan should also include a statement or goal on promoting research training within the organization. This type of education is invaluable for the workforce in general as it increases critical thinking capabilities and sensitizes the workforce on the role of research in the delivery of health care (the promotion of evidence-based practice).

There are a number of ways to develop a research qualified workforce. Some of these are formal such as supporting postgraduate training programs or creating research internships. Ideally, large-scale grants should include a training opportunity for a suitable clinical staff member. This may be in terms of a masters, doctoral or postdoctoral degree. A masters degree usually involves a research component of up to one year. For the Doctor of Philosophy (PhD) degree a substantial piece of research (up to 3 years) is usually undertaken. Postdoctoral degrees give recent PhD graduates an opportunity to continue to work in a supportive environment to develop more advanced skills such as grant writing and the management of research projects. They last up to 5 years. Informal experiential training is another way to develop the clinical workforce. This can occur through work on small projects with the visiting scholars or on larger projects in a junior role with more experienced researchers. Some of the 'dryness' of research training can be overcome by actually doing research that is of interest to the clinician. Research training workshops can also help staff. A program that groups staff into teams and provides mentorship will help small staff-driven projects succeed. These small projects do not necessarily have to fit into your overall research theme or direction (although it is great if they do) because in effect they are providing research training at a beginning level according to the interest of the staff member. These types of studies rarely have sufficient scope or power to produce findings that can endorse a change to practice but can generate enthusiasm for research and prompt staff to join larger studies that have the capacity to produce more robust findings.

▶ **Research governance**

An important aspect of research from a risk management point of view is to ensure that you have the correct governance procedures in place. These need not be onerous but should be allocated as a direct responsibility to an organizational officer. If the organization does not convene an ethics committee, you may wish to consider doing so. Chapters 2 and 4 explain the ethical obligations regarding research and provide links for more information in this area. If you decide not to convene an organizational ethics committee (and many smaller facilities take this path), you need to ensure that the research conducted at your facility has independent ethical review. Small facilities often 'buddy' with larger facilities in this regard. If you intend to use a University Ethics Committee, care needs to be taken that they understand the ethical issues as they relate to patient care and the healthcare facility. If this is your preferred option, it would be wise to ask for a senior member of your organization to participate on the committee.

Your next task is to develop, maintain and promote a searchable database of facility research projects and results. This allows you to track and monitor the research that is happening in your facility. It should include the following details.

---

### Check List: Information required on an organizational research register

☑ Names of all the investigators
☑ Name of the Chief Investigator or the designated contact person
☑ Name of the project
☑ Short (100 words) plain language description of the project
☑ Start and estimated finish date
☑ Funding sources
☑ Progress details (in progress or complete)
☑ Outputs (presentations, conference papers, journal articles)

---

### ▶ Measures of success

Periodic assessment and review of the research program should be undertaken to determine the effectiveness of the research investment for your organization. The usual measures of research quality have centred on grants (inputs) and publications (outputs) with citations (i.e., how often the work is cited in other publications). There is vigorous debate on the usefulness of this approach and research quality measures are being reviewed in the United Kingdom, Australia and New Zealand. Many funding bodies are now moving towards measuring the impact of the research for end users in the community. From an organizational perspective other measures can also be of use. The following list provides you with some of the more common performance indicators used in research including general performance measures and impact indicators.

**Part 3**

---

### ✒ Check List: Research performance indicators

☑ Grants
☑ Invited presentations
☑ Publications
☑ Citations
☑ Patents
☑ Documented clinical practice change from using research findings
☑ Documented changed in policies or processes by incorporation of research findings

---

## ▶ Summary

The primary function of any healthcare facility is as a service provider for a particular population group. In common with universities many also teach students of the healthcare professions. Most facilities, particularly the larger ones, are concerned to contribute to healthcare knowledge by providing high-quality research. In this chapter we have shown you how to address this using a strategic planning approach, that is in step with the large grant rounds provided by government. Once the research direction has been set, building capacity within organizations can be a simple as starting a 'visiting scholars' program, a cost-neutral initiative that can foster good relationships with tertiary partners. Finally, we have considered the management of risk associated with research in major facilities and have provided some simple ways of ensuring you track and evaluate your research program.

## ▶ Reference

ABS (1998). Australian Standard Research Classification (ASRC), Cat. No. 1297.0, ABS, Canberra.

# Doing clinical research: a summary

*Sarah Winch*

Conducting research in busy healthcare facilities requires a strategic focus and a great deal of preparatory work. The rewards for your efforts are the production of findings that have the ability to influence patient care through direct clinical interventions or by improving workforce practices and culture.

A constant theme through this book has been the need to establish strategic teams and to communicate effectively with all stakeholders. Creating a research opportunity that has the capacity to deliver good outcomes for both the researchers and the facility is critical to the success of your endeavours. In Chapter 1 we explained this in terms of framing your research question so that it has a hook and a heart that grabs the attention of clinical or academic partners. The following check list reviews what is needed to ensure your project succeeds.

 **Check List: Summary for project preparation success**

☑ Champion found amongst senior staff
☑ Sponsor available
☑ Research topic addresses organizational needs or research priorities (hook)
☑ Funding or resources are available or will be applied for
☑ Academic partner(s) have necessary research experience
☑ Clinical staff have a broad understanding and commitment to the research topic (heart)
☑ Clinical staff (medical and nursing are committed to the project)
☑ Communication plan developed

**Part 3**

Many researchers find the process of approaching and securing ethical clearance for their work daunting, yet this is an essential part of conducting research. In Chapter 2 we showed you how to identify systematically all of the possible ethical implications of your research. To assist you further, we developed a master proposal template that will prompt you to address the ethical issues associated with conducting research.

Research conducted in nations from different cultures is challenging and requires careful planning in terms of access and language. It is easy to get things wrong, and perhaps cause offence or make a major error in conducting your research. Assess the situation before you leave your own country and consult foreign embassies and travel guidance. If translation into another language is necessary, there are many techniques to ensure that the translations are correct and culturally relevant. Undertaking research with Indigenous populations requires extra work gaining access and permission to conduct the research, and to gain ethical approval. Most countries that have Indigenous populations have government bodies from which special approval and permission have to be sought.

In Chapter 4 we provided the *master proposal* template. When completed, this is invaluable for communication purposes, grant applications and ethics approval. In this chapter we also explained about the risks (for the researcher and the organization) associated with conducting research in terms of legal obligations. This area is becoming increasingly complex and needs regular review by checking with the links that we have provided.

Enhancing recruitment and reducing time wasted in this activity is a key feature of ensuring that your project is successful. When local staff are informed and involved, then they can be keen to assist – and become invaluable team members. Charge nurses who largely co-ordinate the healthcare team are often pivotal in assisting with access as they are particularly knowledgeable about patient populations and profiles, together with healthcare routines and activities.

In Chapter 6 we explained the best ways to use the variety of methods available to collect data in health facilities with both clinical and staff populations. These considerations need to be examined quite closely with both the question and the proposed population to determine with confidence the best way to collect your data for maximum participation and quality that directly affects the worthiness of the findings.

The data collection theme is explored further in Chapter 7 where we explained how to collect data in a systematic fashion. Whether the data be in the form of surveys, tapes, videos or written notes, it needs to be meticulously collected and a system needs to be established to progress the analysis of the data (even if it is an agreed set of meetings with the team).

There are particular considerations that are worthwhile remembering for particular methods to ensure rigour in the process. If there is insufficient detail in the data that has been collected then this will directly affect the cogency of the analysis of the data.

At the completion of the collection and compilation of the data, the process of making sense of what it means can seem overwhelming. It is important that you have considered how you will undertake this task from the beginning, as assumptions made at the beginning will influence the data analysis. Chapter 8 provides some pointers on how you can organize this data ready for the process who have decided for analysis. In addition, suggestions have been made to revisit the initial questions, and also conceptual maps that were developed when you were proposing the research. This can be a useful guide during the interpretation of your research where you need to explain to the wider community why it was important that your research was conducted.

By taking the trouble to publish your findings, you are completing the research loop and adding to the evidence base of healthcare. The Chief Investigator needs to show leadership in this area by ensuring that findings are disseminated in the most appropriate manner for the stage of the research. For example, it is perfectly acceptable for 'work in progress' to be presented as conference papers or posters. To balance the load of writing reports and publications, ensure that all team members take a part in the process. This way the process is not so onerous on one individual and others may learn about the publication process.

We observed in our first chapter that the primary function of any healthcare facility is as a service provider for a particular population group. Yet, most facilities, particularly the larger ones, are concerned to contribute to healthcare knowledge by providing high-quality research. In our final chapter we showed you how to build a rich research environment by using a strategic planning approach. Once the research direction has been set, building capacity within organizations can be a simple as starting a 'visiting scholars' program, a cost neutral initiative that can foster good relationships with tertiary partners. Finally, we have considered the management of risk associated with research in major facilities and have provided some simple ways of ensuring you track and evaluate your research programme.

This book has been written for people like yourself, clinicians, managers or academics who are keen to develop a body of knowledge that will advance their respective disciplines and most importantly, in some way, improve patient care. In this endeavour we are all in agreement! Our aim has been to produce an informative and practical book that will help you

**Part 3**

overcome some of the unforeseen barriers and produce the findings that are worthy of your efforts and those who have supported you and your team including the research participants. We hope with these insights your research plans can become a reality and make a significant contribution to health care in the future through communicating your great work.

# Index